Practice Accounts
Made Easy

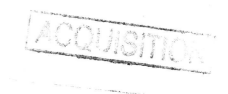

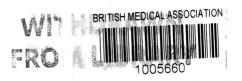

OTHER BOOKS FROM SCION

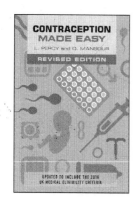

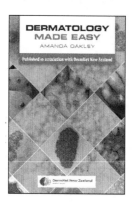

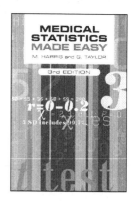

For more details see www.scionpublishing.com

Practice Accounts Made Easy *2nd Edition*

Ann Tudor FCA
Principal – Tudor Healthcare Accountants LLP

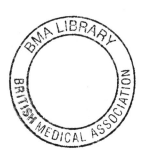

Scion

Scion Publishing Limited

The Old Hayloft, Vantage Business Park, Bloxham Road, Banbury OX16 9UX, UK

www.scionpublishing.com

Important Note from the Publisher

The information contained within this book was obtained by Scion Publishing Ltd from sources believed by us to be reliable. However, while every effort has been made to ensure its accuracy, no responsibility for loss or injury whatsoever occasioned to any person acting or refraining from action as a result of information contained herein can be accepted by the authors or publishers.

Readers are reminded that medicine is a constantly evolving science and while the authors and publishers have ensured that all dosages, applications and practices are based on current indications, there may be specific practices which differ between communities. You should always follow the guidelines laid down by the manufacturers of specific products and the relevant authorities in the country in which you are practising.

Although every effort has been made to ensure that all owners of copyright material have been acknowledged in this publication, we would be pleased to acknowledge in subsequent reprints or editions any omissions brought to our attention.

Registered names, trademarks, etc. used in this book, even when not marked as such, are not to be considered unprotected by law.

Typeset by Phoenix Photosetting, Chatham, Kent, UK

Printed in the UK by 4edge Limited

Contents

Preface to the second edition

The intention of this book is to provide GPs with a straightforward and clear explanation of what makes up their practice accounts and what they should expect to see. It also explains how the figures interact and should be interpreted. It looks at the medical practice from a business perspective to help GPs understand the commercial aspects of their medical activity. Additionally, the book includes explanations of how the UK tax system applies to GPs and considers relevant aspects of the NHS Pension Scheme.

Primary care is currently experiencing significant change as the impact of NHS England's *Five Year Forward View* document, which was published in October 2014, begins to translate into new ways of delivering care and, in particular, addressing the report's emphasis on working at scale. Many GPs are now working either in larger merged practices or in alliances or federations with other GP practices. Additionally, some GPs are working with other healthcare professionals in corporate structures. Understanding the underlying financial structure of a GP practice becomes even more important as these new, more sophisticated groups evolve and become established.

This book is based in part upon a previous publication, *Understanding Practice Accounts*. In *Practice Accounts Made Easy* I have brought that book up to date and extended the content to support GPs and their practice managers, so that they can better evaluate the financial performance of the practice.

To aid understanding, I have created a fictitious (but realistic) set of annual accounts for High Street Medical Practice. The relevant sections of these are appended to each chapter and I refer to them when explaining how accounts work.

I am aware that the names and gender of the doctors used in the examples in this book are not representative of current GP practice; however, the Tudor family dogs would be devastated if they were not included in this way!

Ann Tudor
April 2017

Acknowledgements

My thanks, in particular, go to my colleagues at Tudor Healthcare Accountants for their support and help in writing this book and for keeping the balls juggling whilst I was locked away in writing mode.

I am also grateful to Dr Lachlan Arblaster and Dr Nuzhet A-Ali for checking from a GP perspective that the material in this book made sense and was helpful.

Abbreviations

ACA	Associate Chartered Accountant
AIA	Annual Investment Allowance
AISMA	Association of Independent Specialist Medical Accountants
APMS	Alternative Provider Medical Services
CCG	Clinical commissioning group
CIC	Community Interest Company
CQC	Care Quality Commission
DBS	Disclosure and Barring Service
DDRB	Doctors' and Dentists' Review Body
FCA	Fellow Chartered Accountant
FYA	First year allowance
GMC	General Medical Council
GMS	General Medical Services
HMRC	Her Majesty's Revenue and Customs (Inland Revenue)
LLP	Limited Liability Partnership
MCP	Multispecialty community provider
MPIG	Minimum Practice Income Guarantee
NHSE	NHS England
NI	National Insurance
PCO	Primary Care Organisation
PMS	Personal Medical Services

PSR   Profit sharing ratio
QOF   Quality and Outcomes Framework
SFE   Statement of Financial Entitlements
WDA   Writing-down allowance

Chapter 1

Introduction to practice accounts

What are practice accounts?

Practice accounts are an historic record of the financial performance of the practice. The accounts themselves typically comprise two main pages:

- the profit and loss account, which can also be called the income and expenditure account
- the balance sheet.

The profit and loss account provides the practice with a record of all its income and expenses for a given period. It also provides the GPs in the practice with information about how the practice profit is shared between them so that they can see how much they have earned in any given period (see *Chapter 2: Profit and loss account*).

The balance sheet provides the practice with a record of the value of its assets and liabilities at a given point in time. It also shows each GP their share of those assets (see *Chapter 3: Balance sheet*).

To be fully informative the accounts should also include notes and supplementary information, including benchmark statistics, to help the practice to understand the make-up of the figures in the profit and loss account and balance sheet. These notes will also enable the accounts to be considered analytically to help the practice measure and compare its financial performance.

The accounts will also include a statement to be signed by all partners confirming their agreement to the accounts. This will be a requirement set out in the practice's partnership agreement. This is important, should disputes subsequently arise.

In addition there will be a statement, to be signed by the accountant once the accounts have been agreed and signed by the partners, confirming the basis on which accounts have been prepared.

Why do we need accounts?

For many GPs, the main purpose of accounts is to calculate the profits to be declared on their tax return which is submitted to Her Majesty's Revenue and Customs (HMRC; commonly referred to as the Inland Revenue). This is a fundamental reason for preparing accounts, but it is also important to make use of the information provided by the accounts by using them to look at the practice finances in a more commercial manner.

Whilst providing an historical record of the financial performance of the practice, the accounts are also a useful tool in making financial decisions. For example, the profit and loss account shows the profitability of the practice. If the GPs are earning low profits they can use the profit and loss account to see why this is, and what changes they need to make to improve their profits; for example, by trying to reduce expenditure (see the section on practice statistics in *Chapter 7: Specialist medical accounts*).

Third parties may also want to see the accounts. For example, the bank may want to ensure that the practice is able to repay any loan commitments, or a potential new partner may want to assess the financial situation of the practice. Additionally if a GP is applying for a personal mortgage his lender may wish to see the accounts or will ask the practice accountant for figures from the accounts, and/or from annual tax returns, to support the proof of earnings for their mortgage application.

How often are accounts prepared?

Practice accounts will usually be prepared annually. However, accounts can be produced more often than once a year. For example, if a partner leaves or joins a practice part way through the year, the practice may decide to prepare the accounts for a shorter period up to the date the partner left. This may be directed in the practice's partnership agreement. This will enable the practice accountant to calculate how much money that partner is owed by the practice. It is not essential to do separate accounts when a partner leaves, and some practices choose to save accountancy fees by using a full year's accounts and apportioning the profits on a month by month basis for the periods before and after the partner leaves. This approach can be modified to take into account any major items of income or expenditure before or after the change, to make sure that the allocation of profits is realistic and the apportionment between the partners fair.

Who prepares accounts and why?

On a day-to-day basis the practice manager or a bookkeeper employed by the practice will record all the financial transactions of the practice. Typically they will use an accounts software package to do this. Some products are specifically tailored for use by a GP practice. This information provides the basis for preparing the year-end practice accounts. The more accurate and reliable these records are, the more economically the accountant can prepare the accounts, thus potentially saving fees. This ongoing data can also be used during the accounting year for the practice to review its financial position.

Normally a practice will employ the services of a qualified Chartered Accountant or a Chartered Certified Accountant to produce its accounts and give financial advice. There is no requirement for GPs to have their accounts audited, so the accounts could be produced by someone who is not a qualified accountant. This is because there is only a requirement for the accounts of large limited companies, public limited companies (PLCs) and large limited liability partnerships (LLPs) to be audited. However, it is recommended that the accounts are produced by an independent firm of qualified specialist medical accountants. An accountant without a formal professional qualification who has experience in preparing medical accounts will be more than capable of providing the necessary advice and supporting a practice's needs. However, qualified accountants will be members of a professional body and will be expected to maintain a high standard of ethical and professional conduct which will give a GP a higher level of confidence.

Types of qualification

There are two main types of qualification which an accountant may have, depending on which professional body's route of study they decided to take.

Chartered Accountant

A Chartered Accountant is a qualified accountant who is a member of the Institute of Chartered Accountants in England and Wales. There is also a separate Scottish Institute. Someone who is a Chartered Accountant will have the letters ACA or FCA after their name.

Chartered Certified Accountant

A Chartered Certified Accountant is a qualified accountant who is a member of the Association of Chartered Certified Accountants. Someone who is a Chartered Certified Accountant will have the letters ACCA or FCCA after their name.

In addition to a professional qualification it is generally seen as important to engage the services of an accountant who specialises in medical practice accounts, because this is a complex area and accountants who have a recognised specialism will be best placed to support GP practices.

One specialist quality endorsed group is the Association of Independent Specialist Medical Accountants (AISMA). AISMA members have to act for a minimum number of GP practices. Members are carefully vetted before being granted membership and quality checks are carried out thereafter. They have access to high quality members' training, technical updates and nationwide statistics.

Do accounts have to be prepared in a certain way?

GP practice accounts comprise the profit and loss account and the balance sheet, with supporting notes and schedules. There is no statutory requirement for a specific format for practice accounts. The accounts are prepared from the practice's accounting records. The presentation of accounts will differ between accountants. However, there is a fairly standard layout for the profit and loss account and balance sheet.

For example, in the profit and loss account, income is normally shown at the top of the page, the expenses are shown next, with the net profit at the bottom. Illustrations for the various sections of the accounts are included throughout this book. The more detail which appears in the accounts, the easier it is for the GPs in the practice to understand their finances. Specialist medical accountants will supply comprehensive information specific to the needs of a GP practice; in particular, breaking down the separate income headings to reflect the types of income the practice receives, e.g. global sum, enhanced services and Quality and Outcomes Framework (QOF) (see *Chapter 8: How GPs get paid*).

Management of the accounts process in the practice

The practice manager usually has overall responsibility for the day-to-day financial management in a GP practice. Their responsibilities will include paying bills and salaries, making sure timely claims for income are made and paid, monitoring cash flow and generally safeguarding and administering the finance function.

The practice manager may be supported by a bookkeeper or other administrative staff. The bookkeeping is sometimes outsourced and many specialist medical accountants offer an outsourcing service to support their clients.

It works very well when one of the partners in the practice has a responsibility for practice finances, working with the practice manager, supporting them and providing a sounding board.

Chapter 2
Profit and loss account

The profit and loss account shows the income that the practice has received minus the various expenses (which are also referred to as overheads) incurred in running the practice for a given time period. The expenses are deducted from the income to give the net profit for that period. An example of the profit and loss account for High Street Medical Practice is provided at the end of this chapter.

Why is it important?

The profit and loss account is important because it shows the profitability of the practice. Profit means how much money has been earned from the day-to-day activities of running the practice.

- GPs are conducting a business, and the main object of a business is usually to maximise profits.
- The profit and loss account can be used as a starting point for financial analysis of the business, which can contribute to planning for the future management of the business.
- The profits of the practice will need to be calculated, because this will need to be declared on the practice's self-assessment tax return for HMRC. These data then feed across to the individual partners' tax returns to establish their taxable income from which their tax liabilities are calculated (see *Chapter 9: Taxation*).

- New partners thinking about joining a practice will be interested in the profitability of the practice, because this will give them an indication of their likely earnings, from which they can decide whether or not they wish to join the practice as a partner. Typically they would ask if they can show the accounts to their own accountant to obtain independent advice.
- The practice's bank manager will also be interested in the profitability of the practice, so that he can take a view as to whether the GPs are earning enough income to continue to repay any debts that they may have with the bank.
- If a GP is seeking a personal mortgage or loan their lender will require accounts information to support details of their earnings.

> **Profit and loss**
>
> The profit and loss account (sometimes known as the income and expenditure account) shows the income, expenses and net profit for a given time period.

Accounting period

The profit and loss account covers the practice's accounting period. The accounting period will normally be a 12-month period to its year-end date, with the practice's year-end date normally being decided when the practice commences trading; it is usually 12 months after this date. In the example provided in this chapter, the practice's year-end is 30 June. This means that the initial partners probably commenced trading as a practice sometime in the past on 1 July and so the accounting period runs from 1 July to 30 June the following year.

If the accounting period does not cover 12 months, the accounts should clearly state what period they do cover. This would normally be shown on the front page of the accounts, for example 'For the period from 1 July to 31 December'.

When you start a practice you do not need to run your first accounts for 12 months and this is the time to seek advice from a specialist medical accountant as to what might be the best year-end going forward. There are a number of considerations.

The usual recommendation is to tie into the NHS year which runs to 31 March. Many practices use this as their year-end so that it is more straightforward to work out what is owed for NHS services that have been delivered by the practice, but for which the practice has not yet been paid (see *Chapter 3: Balance sheet*).

The last day of March is generally a favoured year-end for income tax and superannuation, because it provides a close correlation to the tax and pension annual cycles. (see *Chapter 9: Taxation*).

It should be noted that accounting periods can be different to the tax year, which runs from 6 April to 5 April the following year (see *Chapter 9: Taxation*).

Comparative figures

The accounts should also include comparative figures from the previous accounting period. In the example shown at the end of this chapter, the profit and loss account shows the figures for 12 months to 30 June 2016 and also the previous 12 months to 30 June 2015. This allows the practice to compare the current year's figures to those of the previous year and identify any variances that may need investigation.

In the example, staff costs for the year ended 30 June 2016 are £660,655 and for the year ended 30 June 2015 the costs were £636,527. There has therefore been an increase of £24,128 (£660,655 minus £636,527). The GPs in the practice should consider why there has been an increase, to justify the amounts included in the accounts, and to help them to achieve a better understanding of what is going on in their business. For instance, they should work out the financial impact of any pay rises, any changes in the people they employ and their relative pay costs, or the cost of covering any sick leave for a member of staff.

Income

The income that the practice has earned will be shown at the top of the profit and loss account. Different accountants will present the income in different ways (see *Chapter 7: Specialist Medical Accounts*).

The example shows five headings for income:
- General Medical Services (GMS) or Personal Medical Services (PMS) income
- Reimbursement of expenses
- Other NHS income
- Other non-NHS income
- Dispensing income.

An analysis of these headings is shown separately on additional pages called 'Schedules' or 'Notes' (in this case, Notes 2, 8, 9, 10 and 11). The income headings above include income from the following sources:
- GMS or PMS income – this is the total figure for the income earned from the practice's GMS or PMS contract for the care of the practice's patients (see *Chapter 8: How GPs get paid*).
- Reimbursement of expenses – this is the total figure for the reimbursements the practice has received towards the cost of running the practice (see *Chapter 8: How GPs get paid*).
- Other NHS income – this is the total value of other income from NHS activity, additional to the mainstream GMS or PMS contract income (see *Chapter 8: How GPs get paid*).
- Other non-NHS income – this is any income that the practice has earned from other activities; for example, reports for insurance companies, medico-legal work or other services, such as hosting services.
- Dispensing income – this income comes from prescriptions for drugs administered in the practice, such as flu vaccines. For a dispensing practice this would also include dispensing prescriptions to the practice's dispensing patients (see *Chapter 8: How GPs get paid*).

The example accounts show that the practice has earned total income of £1,147,435 for the 12 months to 30 June 2016. In the previous 12 months the practice earned total income of £1,136,466. Total income can also be called gross income, where gross means before taking off any expenses. The words 'total' and 'gross' are interchangeable in this context.

Grossing up principle

Total or gross income is income which has not been reduced by taking off any related expenditure. In medical practices it is important to show total income and total expenditure separately without netting one off against the other. Netting off might be applied when you claim a reimbursement for the purchase of a specific item or service so that overall the transaction is nil, for example £1000 in and £1000 out. Netting off means you don't include either transaction in your accounts because it has no overall impact on the profit.

An example of a situation where netting off might have seemed the appropriate way to deal with transactions would be the income and expenditure through the prescribing incentive scheme. In recent years practices have been able to claim money through this scheme. The scheme represents money saved through adopting CCG prescribing recommendations. Claims are made for specific purchases of equipment, facilities or service provision which will improve clinical services and/or experience for patients. The income claimed covers the amount paid for, for example, the equipment purchased and, therefore, exactly matches the expenditure. In the accounts there could be a view that because the transactions cancel one another out financially they have no impact on the practice's profit and, therefore, neither the income nor expenditure should be shown in the profit and loss account.

This would not be the correct accounting treatment in medical practice accounts, where the 'grossing up' principle should be applied. This means that the whole of the income from the prescribing incentive scheme should be included in the practice income and the whole of the payment for the related equipment purchase or service provision should be shown in the practice expenses, under the appropriate heading.

Another example of grossing up which may not be as obvious is the situation where the CCG has a contract for service delivery for all practices in its control. Typically this might be the clinical waste contract. The CCG will pay for the clinical waste disposal directly to the contractor who undertakes this service. Practices will be notified of their share of such payments by their CCG, and they need to make sure that this information is given to their accountant who will then include the clinical waste cost as an expense and also include as income the same figure as a reimbursement by the CCG for that expense.

GP accounts are scrutinised and become part of national statistics. Data are collated and published by NHS Digital. By adopting the grossing up principle practices can more clearly demonstrate the investment of their income into health-related or support services for their clinical work. Additionally, comparisons within the statistics are recognised on the same basis.

In addition, the Doctors' and Dentists' Review Body (DDRB) scrutinises practice accounts sampled from self-assessment tax returns provided by HMRC to enable it to make pay recommendations to the Department of Health. This review includes looking at the relationship between gross income and net profits. Minimising the percentage retained by GPs as profit from the gross payments to practices, which is achieved by adopting the grossing up principle, has historically been a useful tool in pay negotiations.

By way of example, let's say the gross income of a practice is £800,000. This includes business rates paid by the CCG of £25,000. The expenses of the practice total £500,000, which includes as a payment the £25,000 business rates. The net profit is £300,000 (£800,000 less £500,000). The net profit as a percentage of gross income is 37.5% (£300,000 divided by £800,000 multiplied by 100). If the £25,000 was excluded from gross income because it had been netted off the expense, this would make the gross income £775,000. The net profit would be the same because expenses would have been reduced by £25,000. The net profit as a percentage of income is now 38.71% (£300,000 divided by £775,000 multiplied by 100).

As can be seen from this example, when a practice adopts the grossing up principle it appears to have retained a lower percentage of its gross income as personal profit, which helps correctly recognise the GP practice's financial position. This in turn will mean that GPs are properly represented when negotiating pay rises and it also helps to appropriately present their financial situation in the media.

Overheads / expenses

Overheads are the expenses that are incurred in the day-to-day running of the practice; for example, the staff costs cover the salaries for the practice staff. In this example, the expenses are categorised, with more information and breakdowns in the notes accompanying the accounts. Different accountants may present the expenses in different ways.

> **Overheads / expenses**
>
> These words mean the same thing. Some accountants may use the word overheads, others may use the word expenses.

The example shows the practice incurred expenses of £829,296 for the 12 months to 30 June 2016. The comparative expenses for the 12 months to 30 June 2015 were £808,722.

Net profit

The income less the expenses gives the practice's net profit for the period. This is the net income the practice has earned after paying its expenses. The net profit is important as it shows the profitability of the practice. In this example, the practice earned a net profit of £318,139 for the 12 months to 30 June 2016. The comparative net profit for the 12 months to 30 June 2015 was £327,744.

Net profit or gross profit

Accountants refer to gross profit and net profit.

Gross profit. For a trading business which buys goods at one price and then sells the same goods at a higher price, the difference between the two represents a profit which is known as the gross profit. This is the profit on the sale of these goods. For example, if I purchase an item for £10 and then sell the same item for £15, the gross profit would be £5.

This part of the profit and loss account is shown separately to the main profit and loss account and starts with the income received from the sale of these items. The cost of these items (known as 'cost of sales') is then deducted. The difference is the gross profit. The only aspect of a GP practice accounts for which the calculation of the gross profit is relevant is for dispensing activity. The practice buys drugs and the cost of the drugs would be shown as the 'cost of sales'; these drugs would then be dispensed, which would generate income. The difference between the income and cost of sales is the gross profit.

Dispensing	2016	2015
	£	£
Dispensing fees and allowance paid to cover the cost of drugs	45,636	42,788
Cost of purchasing dispensed items	32,459	30,980
Gross profit on dispensing	13,177	11,808
Percentage return	28.87%	27.60%

Dispensing fees for administering the dispensing activity are often shown separately to the allowance paid to cover the cost of the drugs.

The profit and loss account otherwise includes all other income received less the overheads of the practice, which would conclude with the overall net profit of the practice.

Net profit. The net profit is the final profit that the business has made, after deducting all the expenses incurred in running the business.

The net profit is the amount which is then shared by the partners to give their individual earnings for the year (see *Chapter 4: Profit allocation*).

If the partners want to increase the amount that they earn, they need to increase the profitability of the practice. To increase profitability a practice needs to increase the income earned and/or reduce the practice expenses incurred.

Notes to the accounts

The accounts themselves are two pages, the profit and loss account and the balance sheet. All other pages and information are subordinate to these pages. On these two pages there will be reference to 'Notes' or 'Schedules'; the two words are used interchangeably. These are additional pages, which provide further information and explanations for the figures in the profit and loss or balance sheet. In our example accounts, the supplementary information is contained in notes which follow the balance sheet in the accounts pack. The 'accounts pack' is the description for all accounts information, including any benchmarking or statistical information.

Publication of earnings

From 1 April 2015 there has been a contractual requirement for practices to publish the mean earnings for all GPs in the practice on the practice website. The published data need to include the number of full- and part-time GPs included in the calculation.

High Street Medical Practice
Profit and Loss Account
Year ended 30 June 2016

	Notes	Y/E 30.06.2016 £	Y/E 30.06.2015 £
Practice income			
GMS/PMS income	2	995,269	987,378
Reimbursement of expenses	8	50,550	48,550
Other NHS income	9	36,700	36,100
Other non-NHS income	10	19,280	21,650
Dispensing income	11	45,636	42,788
TOTAL INCOME		1,147,435	1,136,466
Practice expenditure			
Dispensing costs	11	32,459	30,980
Medical expenses	12	30,035	27,425
Premises expenses	13	33,443	41,880
Staff costs	14	660,655	636,527
Administrative expenses	15	17,133	13,836
Finance charges	16	7,676	8,634
Other expenses	17	8,455	8,890
Depreciation	18	1,440	1,550
Employers' superannuation	19	38,000	39,000
TOTAL EXPENDITURE		829,296	808,722
Net profit for the year		318,139	327,744

The note numbers in the example are expanded on in *Chapter 7: Specialist medical accounts.*

Chapter 3

Balance sheet

The profit and loss account shows the income and expenses for the accounting period, and usually covers a 12-month period. In contrast, the balance sheet shows the values of the assets and liabilities on a single day. Hence, the balance sheet represents a snapshot of the practice's finances on that day. This day will usually be the practice's year-end date. There is an example of a balance sheet at the end of this chapter.

Assets and liabilities

Assets are items or amounts that the practice owns or are amounts of money which are owed to the practice. For example, if the partners own the surgery premises, then this is an asset. The money in the bank account is also an asset. The assets can be divided into 'fixed' and 'current' assets. Fixed assets represent long-term assets (often the premises plus any equipment, furnishings, etc. which may have been bought by the practice). Current assets represent short-term assets (such as cash).

Liabilities are amounts that the practice owes. For example, the mortgage for the premises is a liability, as it is owed to the lender.

There are two halves to the balance sheet. The top half lists the value of all the assets and liabilities of the practice and arrives at a total of the assets less the liabilities. The bottom half shows how much each partner owns of these assets. The partners' share of assets can be shown as capital and current accounts. The value of the assets and liabilities (top half of the balance sheet) is the same value as the capital and current accounts (bottom half of the balance sheet) – hence the term 'balance' sheet.

Capital and current accounts

The terms 'capital account' and 'current account' can be interchangeable and refer to the wealth of the practice. The total of a partner's capital and current accounts is the amount of money that a partner has invested in the practice and it will be this amount that a partner is entitled to be paid when they leave the practice. In the example balance sheet, the capital accounts represent each partner's share of the net equity in the surgery property (the value of the freehold property is £400,000 less the balance owing on the property loan which is £250,000, giving a net value of £150,000). However, not all accountants identify capital accounts in this way. Some show the capital account as a fixed amount which the partners have agreed. In the example balance sheet the current accounts, which represent the partners' undrawn profits, are £21,060 at 30 June 2016, compared to £17,850 at 30 June 2015 (see *Chapter 6: Capital and current accounts* for more information on this aspect of the balance sheet).

The balance sheet should also include comparative figures showing the value of the assets at the previous year-end date. In the example shown in this chapter, the balance sheet is a snapshot of the value of assets and liabilities at 30 June 2016, and the comparative shows the value at 30 June 2015.

Fixed assets

Fixed assets are those assets that are long term and have a lifespan of more than 12 months. These include the surgery premises (if owned by the partners in the practice), fixtures and fittings, office and medical equipment, etc. Fixed assets are divided into tangible and intangible assets:

- **Tangible assets** will be the premises (if owned), fixtures, fittings, and office and medical equipment. Tangible means the assets physically exist – they can be touched. (See *Chapter 5: Fixed assets* for further information and an explanation on how tangible assets are valued and depreciated.)
- **Intangible assets** are assets which do not have a physical, tangible existence; for example, goodwill. Because a medical practice cannot buy or sell goodwill relating to core NHS services, intangible assets relating to goodwill will rarely feature in medical practice accounts. An example of an intangible asset that may feature is an investment such as shares bought by the practice in a company which provides the structure for a federation of practices. Alternatively, the cost of shares may be described as investments in the balance sheet.

Net property equity

This is the difference between the value of the premises and the balance outstanding on the mortgage. If a practice is in negative equity, it means that its mortgage is higher than the value of the premises. Negative equity is comparatively rare in a medical practice.

Net equity

This is the difference between all of the assets and liabilities in the practice balance sheet. If a practice is in negative equity, it means that its liabilities are higher than its assets, probably because the partners have taken out more in their drawings than the practice has accumulated in annual profits. Such practices will usually be supported by a bank overdraft to fund this overdrawing, and their situation will need careful monitoring to control the cash flow and thereby manage the bank overdraft going forward. Clearly the ideal scenario is positive equity!

Current assets

Current assets are short-term assets which can be turned into cash in the next 12 months. These include stock of drugs, debtors and bank funds. The value of these will change from day to day. For example, the money in the bank account will change due to income being received and overheads being paid.

Current assets will be made up of the following elements:

Stock

This is the value of the stock of drugs at the year-end. Normally the drugs left at the year-end will be listed and counted and then valued at their cost price. In this example, there is stock of £1,575 left at the year-end. A dispensing practice would have a more significant stock level, but most practices will have a small stock of dressings and drugs which, for instance, might be required for a patient who is on a course of treatment. These drugs are called personally administered items.

Where a practice holds a stock of other consumables, such as toners for printers, these should also be valued and included in the stock figure on the balance sheet if they are of significant value.

Debtors

Debtors comprise money that is owed from third parties to the practice. The practice will have completed work within the accounting period but will not yet have received payment for it. For example, certain enhanced services may be paid on submission of a claim by the practice. In this example, the debtors are £44,500, which means that the practice is owed this amount of money and it should be received in the bank account after the year-end, i.e. after 30 June 2016.

Prepayments

These represent expenses that have been prepaid for a particular period. For example, a practice may pay its building and contents insurance in January 2016 to cover the whole year up to 31 December

2016. If its year-end is 30 June 2016, it would have paid from 1 July 2016 to 31 December 2016 in advance. The amount for that period would be treated as being prepaid. In the example balance sheet prepayments at 30 June 2016 total £863.

Bank balance

This will be the reconciled bank balance at the year-end. Reconciled means the balance at the year-end less any cheques that were written in the accounting period but which had not cleared the bank at the year-end, and any money paid into the account by the practice but not shown on the bank statement at the time (because the amount was being processed through the bank clearing system when the reconciliation process was being undertaken). If the bank account is overdrawn this will be shown under current liabilities. A bank account that is overdrawn means that the practice owes money to the bank. (Note that this is represented as a liability, rather than being in brackets under current assets.) In this example, the reconciled bank balance is £3,990 overdrawn and appears as a current liability.

Cash in hand

This will be the amount of cash that is left in the petty cash tin at the year-end. In this example, the amount of cash left at 30 June 2016 is £210.

Current liabilities

Current liabilities are amounts that are owed to a third party at the year-end date and are payable within 12 months. They are usually made up of the following elements.

Creditors and accruals

This is the amount owed to third parties at the year-end; for example, drugs purchased during the accounting period, but not paid for by the time of the year-end. In this example, the creditors outstanding at 30 June 2016 are £23,458.

Creditors are amounts owed for which the practice holds invoices for the purchase of the goods or services bought. This includes amounts due to HMRC for the income tax and National Insurance contributions deducted from staff pay which then has to be paid to HMRC. This is always paid in the month following the deduction.

Accruals are estimates for amounts owed where the practice knows it has received a service but hasn't yet had an invoice. An example of an accrual is the amount owed to the practice accountant for preparing the practice accounts. Because this is an ongoing assignment at the time when the accounts are being prepared, an invoice has probably not yet been sent to the practice, so an estimate or a figure based on a quote will be included as an accrual.

Another example is where an expense covers a period of time which includes some weeks before the year-end, but the cost will not be invoiced / charged and paid until after the full period of time has elapsed after the year-end, such as quarterly loan interest on a bank loan account. If at the year-end it is one month since the last interest payment then an accrual for two-thirds (the next 2 months of the quarter) of the next payment needs to be included when the accounts are prepared.

Bank overdraft

See 'bank balance' section above.

Bank loan

If the practice has a short-term bank loan, the outstanding balance due at the year-end would probably be shown under current liabilities. However, it would not be shown as a current liability if it was a longer-term loan with, say, five or more years to repayment. For example, the mortgage for the premises would not be shown as a current liability because this is a long-term loan. The reason for this is that current liabilities are those liabilities which are payable within 12 months, whereas a mortgage is likely to be repayable over a much longer period, so would normally be shown as a long-term liability. The practice accountant may decide to show the instalments due in the next 12 months as a current liability and the balance of the loan as a long-term liability.

In this example, the bank loan is referred to as 'property loan' and appears under long-term loans. The amount owing at 30 June 2016 is £250,000.

Total assets

The total of the current liabilities is deducted from the current assets to give the net current assets. In this example the total of the current liabilities is £27,448, which is deducted from the total current assets of £47,148 to give the net current assets of £19,700.

The net current assets are then added to the fixed assets. In this example, the net assets of £19,700 are added to the total fixed assets of £401,360 to give the total assets (less current liabilities) of £421,060.

The long-term liabilities, comprising the property loan of £250,000, are then deducted to arrive at net assets for the practice of £171,060.

So what does the figure of £171,060 mean to a practice? In effect, it is the amount of money that the partners would have left if they sold all their assets and paid off all their liabilities at the date the balance sheet had been prepared.

If the partners decided to dissolve the practice on 30 June 2016 and sold the property for £400,000, then paid off the mortgage of £250,000, the net amount remaining of £150,000 would be paid into the bank account and increase the bank balance by £150,000. If the fixtures, fittings and equipment were sold for the value on the balance sheet, the bank account would increase by a further £1,360. The practice would return its stock to the suppliers and receive £1,575 which would further increase the bank balance. It would receive payments from its debtors (money owed to it) and this would increase the bank account by £45,363. It would pay the petty cash balance of £210 into the bank account. It would have to pay its creditors (money owed by the practice), which would reduce the bank balance by £23,458. After all of these transactions the bank account balance would be £171,060. This would not simply be split equally between the partners, but would be split depending on who owned the assets.

Who owns the assets?

The bottom half of the balance sheet shows the ownership of the practice by way of capital accounts and current accounts. Each partner's share of the wealth is shown in their individual capital account and current account. This is their investment in the practice and would be the cash to which they are entitled if they were to leave the practice, or if the practice had ceased on 30 June 2016 (see *Chapter 6: Capital and current accounts* for a further explanation).

In the example of this balance sheet at 30 June 2016, Dr Archie has a balance on his capital account of £75,000 and has a balance on his current account of £4,160. Therefore, if he left the practice at 30 June 2016 and sold his share of the property, he would be owed £79,160 (£75,000 + £4,160). If he left the practice, but kept his share of the property as an investment, then he would be owed £4,160. He would not be paid his capital account because this represents his share of the equity in the property and, as he is not selling his share of the property, he is not entitled to his share of equity.

If Dr Archie had left the practice on 30 June 2015 then the position would have been different because at that time his current account was overdrawn by £3,000 (the brackets round the value show this to be a negative value). His capital account balance was £65,000. Therefore, if he had left the practice on 30 June 2015 and sold his share of the property, he would be owed £62,000 (£65,000 − £3,000). If he had left the practice, but kept his share of the property as an investment, then he would have owed £3,000 to the practice to repay his overdrawn current account.

High Street Medical Practice
Balance Sheet
As at 30 June 2016

	Notes	As at 30 June 2016 £	As at 30 June 2016 £	As at 30 June 2015 £	As at 30 June 2015 £
Fixed assets	20				
Freehold property			400000		400,000
Fixtures, fittings and equipment			1,360		1,500
			401,360		401,500
Current assets					
Stock of drugs		1,575		1,250	
Debtors		44,500		40,841	
Prepayments		863		535	
Cash in hand		210		150	
		47,148		42,776	
Current liabilities					
Creditors and accruals		23,458		24,571	
Bank overdraft		3,990		1,855	
		27,448		26,426	
Net current assets			19,700		16,350
			421,060		417,850
Long-term loans					
Property loan			250,000		270,000
			171,060		147,850
Represented by: -					
Capital accounts	23				
Dr Archie		75,000		65,000	
Dr Bertie		37,500		32,500	
Dr Sidney		37,500	150,000	32,500	130,000
Current accounts	24				
Dr Archie		4,160		(3,000)	
Dr Bertie		7,700		12,000	
Dr Sidney		7,000		8,850	
Dr Percy		2,200	21,060	–	17,850
			171,060		147,850

Chapter 4
Profit allocation

The partners in the practice are entitled to a share of profits. This is the net income they have earned for the period. The profit allocation shows how the practice's net profit for the period is shared amongst the partners. There is an example profit allocation at the end of this chapter.

Prior allocation

The profits of the practice are shared according to the profit sharing ratios in force during the relevant accounting period. However, there may be some income or expenses which are not shared in the profit sharing ratios. This income would need to be allocated to the relevant partner before the balance of profits is shared amongst the partners. An example of a type of income which might be prior allocated through this mechanism would be seniority. Most practices allocate seniority to the partner to whom it relates.

Profit sharing ratios

The profit sharing ratios (PSRs) are the ratios in which a partnership shares the net profit.

Examples of prior allocations include the following:

Property-related income and expenses

- **Notional and/or cost rent income.** This income should only be allocated to the partners who own the surgery premises. If all the partners own the premises, it may be owned in different proportions to the PSR. Therefore, this income would be allocated in the proportions that the partners own the premises. For example, a three partner practice may split profits in the ratio of 40:40:20, but they may own the property equally and, therefore, the property-related income and expenditure would be shared equally and not in the ratio 40:40:20.

> **Notional / cost rent**
>
> Practices need premises to work from and are therefore eligible for reimbursements which relate to renting or owning their premises.
>
> If the practice owns its premises it will either be reimbursed on a cost rent or notional rent basis (see *Chapter 8: How GPs get paid* for more information).

- **Mortgage interest.** As this expense relates to the interest on the mortgage for the premises, it should be allocated to the partners who own the surgery premises and in the proportions that they own it. Because this is an expense, it should be deducted from the partners' shares of profits, and will be shown in brackets.

In the example profit allocation provided, at the start of the year the property is owned by the three GPs who are the partners in the practice at that time, in the following proportions: Dr Archie 50%, Dr Bertie 25% and Dr Sidney 25%. Dr Percy joins the practice as a partner from 1 January 2016 and by 30 June 2016 has not bought a share of the surgery property. Therefore the income (notional / cost rent) and related expense (mortgage interest), are shared in the property sharing ratio 50:25:25 between the three property-owning partners.

Prior shared income

- **Seniority.** Seniority is paid to the practice to reward partners for their service to the NHS. The amount the practice receives depends on the number of years each partner has worked in the NHS (see *Chapter 8: How GPs get paid*). As mentioned earlier, because this income is related to the individual partners' years of service, it is usually allocated to the partners that it relates to and not shared in the PSR. In the example shown in this chapter, Dr Archie has £5,500 of seniority as a prior allocation, Dr Bertie £3,500 and Dr Sidney £1,000. This income is paid to the individual partners in addition to their share of the rest of the practice profits.

- **Internal locums.** Where a partner in the practice works extra sessions to cover for others in the practice they will probably be paid separately for this work at locum sessional rates or at a sessional rate agreed between the partners. The partner doing this extra work will be paid from the practice bank account, in the same way that a locum would be paid. However, the payment to the partner has a different accounting treatment to a payment to an external locum. The partner is treated as having extra income from the practice equal to the locum payment. This allocation has the effect of reducing the overall net profit which is divisible between the partners, because it is taken out of that profit and given to the partner who has done the work before the remaining profit is allocated between all partners. Therefore the profit is reduced just as it would have been if the payment had been made to an external locum, because a payment to a locum would have been shown as an expense in the profit and loss account and as such would have reduced the practice profit for allocation to the partners. Dr Archie undertook extra sessions and was paid £500 as an internal locum for this work and Dr Sidney and Dr Percy were each paid an extra £200 for internal locum work. This is referred to as 'other apportionments' in the example of a profit allocation.

Prior shared expenses

- **Personal expenses.** Expenditure in the practice is, in the main, paid out of the practice bank account and relates to the practice as a whole. However, there are some expenses which the individual partners will pay from their personal bank accounts but which relate to the costs of carrying out their work as a partner in a practice. Typical examples are car running costs, mobile phones, personal IT equipment and consumables. These types of expenditure involve an element of personal choice (e.g. what car you drive) and it is fairer for this type of expenditure to be paid for by the partner who is incurring the cost. To enable the partners to obtain tax relief on this expenditure, it must be included as a practice expense on the partnership's self-assessment tax return for HMRC and in many practices the expenses are included in the accounts as a first step towards the necessary HMRC disclosure. This means total transparency in claims between the partners, all of whom are responsible for the accuracy of the figures included in the partnership self-assessment tax return. Some accountants do not include personal expenses in the accounts, but they will nevertheless be included as part of the practice expenditure figures in the partnership tax return, because this is the mechanism whereby tax relief is obtained on these expenses.

The expenses paid by a partner need to be set off against their personal profit and not profit shared, so that when a partner has paid an expense themselves they personally get the tax relief on this expenditure. This is achieved through the prior allocation mechanism, by including each individual partner's expenses as a deduction against their profit. In the example Dr Archie's expenses were £3,000, Dr Bertie's £2,000, Dr Sidney's £2,500 and Dr Percy's £800.

- **Employer's superannuation.** A self-employed GP pays employee and employer superannuation contributions and may also pay added years or buy additional NHS pension benefits. The employer's superannuation has been paid to the practice as part of the GMS global sum payments or the PMS baseline payments. Therefore many accountants show the employer's superannuation cost as a deduction from profits so that the net profit then excludes this cost. There is an alternative accounting treatment, adopted by some accountants, which is not to take the employer's superannuation out of the net profit, but to leave it as part of the income with no expense deducted in the profit and loss account (see *Chapter 10: NHS Pension Scheme* for more information on how superannuation works in practice accounts).

Where the employer's superannuation is included as a practice expense, this should also appear as a deduction in the profit allocation to ensure that this cost is allocated to the partners, because it relates to them individually. Because superannuation contributions are based on superannuable income, this will differ from one partner to another. This is the case even where the core practice profits are shared equally, because it is very unlikely that personal expenses will be exactly the same for each partner. Thus, partners' superannuable income will inevitably differ. Therefore the related cost of the superannuation contributions will differ and so there is a need to reflect each individual GP's cost in the prior allocation section of the profit sharing calculation.

Profits shared in profit sharing ratio

Once the prior allocations have been calculated, the balance of profits will be shared in the PSR (profit sharing ratio). The PSR reflects the amount of time each partner spends in the practice and the contribution each partner makes to the practice activities. The PSR can be calculated based on the number of sessions each partner does, or whether they are full-time or part-time. It may include an element of reward for management or other additional responsibilities. All partners should agree the PSR at the start of each accounting year. This would usually be recorded as part of the partnership agreement. However, the PSR may change from year to year because partners may decide to alter the number of sessions they work, and any changes should be formally recorded as a note or memorandum, signed by all the partners, which should be kept with the partnership agreement.

During the year there may be changes in the PSR. For example, a full-time partner may decide to reduce their hours to part-time, a partner may leave the practice, or a new partner may join during the year.

When these events occur the PSR will need to be revised, agreed and documented, as suggested above, to reflect these changes.

Where there is a change in PSR, the profits earned before and after the change need to be apportioned appropriately. This is generally done by assuming that profits accrue evenly throughout the year. However, where there is income or expenditure specific to the period before or after the change in PSR, this needs to be factored in so that the profit for each period is realistic and representative. Sometimes, particularly where the PSR changes because a partner has left or joined a practice in the accounting period, two sets of accounts may be drawn up. One set will cover the period from the start of the year to the date the partner joins or leaves and the second accounts will cover the rest of the accounting year. This will involve additional accounting costs but may be the only way to be fair in more complex situations.

In this example, Drs Archie, Bertie and Sidney shared profits equally up to 31 December 2015. Dr Percy joined as a partner on 1 January 2016 and the revised PSRs were 4:6:8:6. This reflects Dr Percy joining and Dr Archie reducing his sessions to four a week (effectively going to half-time in a wind-down to retirement) and also Dr Bertie reducing to six sessions, i.e. three-quarter time. Dr Percy works six sessions.

It has been common practice that when a new partner joins a partnership they do not receive a full share of profits. Initially, they might earn between 80% and 90% parity (parity meaning on a par with their fellow partners so that all partners are paid at the same rate for the sessions they work in the practice). However, this arrangement is becoming less frequent. More often a prospective new partner will work as an employee or partner on a fixed share (i.e. a specified amount) in the same way that a fixed agreed salary would be paid to an employee, during their probationary period, which is usually for an initial six months. This is referred to as a mutual assessment period when either the new GP or the partners in the practice can, if applicable, decide that the arrangement is not working and the probationary GP will not go forward to full partnership.

If the six-month trial has been successful, the new partner becomes a full profit sharing partner with the colleagues in the practice. This can also be referred to as a full equity partner.

In the example, the total profits for the year are £318,139. An amount of £25,878 has been prior allocated as expenditure to the partners, leaving a balance of £344,017 (£318,139 + £25,878) to be shared in the PSR. Because there are changes in the ratios during the year, the balance needs to be split into the different periods, as follows:

- **The first period.** This is from the start of the accounting year to the date of the first change, i.e. the six months from 1 July 2015 to 31 December 2015. Because profits are assumed to accrue evenly month by month, the amount of profit for this period is calculated as 6 months divided by 12 months, i.e. 0.5. The balance of profits of £344,017 is multiplied by 0.5. This gives a profit figure for the 6 months of £172,009, which is then split in the PSR for this period (8:8:8).
- **The second period.** This is from 1 January 2016 to 30 June 2016 and again profits would need to be calculated and shared, based on the relevant PSR (4:6:8:6).

For each partner their prior allocation plus their share of the balance is added together to give their total share of profits for the period. In this example:

- Dr Archie has received a total share of profits of £87,353. This is made up of £1,349 (prior allocation) + £57,336 + £28,668.
- Dr Bertie has received £92,663. This is made up of a deduction of −£7,675 (prior allocation) + £57,336 + £43,002.
- Dr Sidney has received £102,614. This is made up of a deduction of −£12,059 (prior allocation) + £57,336 + £57,336.
- Dr Percy has received £35,509. This is made up of a deduction of −£7,493 (prior allocation) + £43,002.

The partner's share of profits, after adjustments for tax purposes, is the start point for their tax and superannuation calculations.

Adjustments to profits for tax

Frequently GPs question why their profits from the profit allocation in the accounts do not match the profit figure on their tax return. This is because for tax purposes, adjustments may need to be made to the calculated profits. This is because some income or expenses may not be allowable for tax purposes. For example, depreciation of the assets is shown as an expense in the profit and loss account, but depreciation is not allowed as a deductible expense for tax. Capital allowances can be claimed on the assets instead of depreciation. The reason for this is that depreciation rates are usually decided by the accountants, whereas the rates for capital allowances are set by tax legislation (see *Chapter 9: Taxation*).

High Street Medical Practice
Profit Allocation
Year ended 30 June 2016

Allocated as follows: -		Total £	Dr Archie £	Dr Bertie £	Dr Sidney £	Dr Percy £
Notional rent		32,000	16,000	8,000	8,000	–
Mortgage interest		(7,478)	(3,739)	(1,870)	(1,870)	–
Seniority		10,000	5,500	3,500	1,000	–
Protection insurance		(15,000)	(4,286)	(4,286)	(4,286)	(2,143)
Personal expenses		(8,300)	(3,000)	(2,000)	(2,500)	(800)
Superannuation		(38,000)	(9,627)	(11,020)	(12,603)	(4,750)
Other apportionments		900	500	–	200	200
		(25,878)	1,349	(7,675)	(12,059)	(7,493)
Balance	01.07.2015 to 31.12.2015 8:8:8	172,009	57,336	57,336	57,336	–
	01.01.2016 to 30.06.2016 4:6:8:6	172,009	28,668	43,002	43,002	43,002
Year ended 30.06.2016		318,139	87,353	92,663	102,614	35,509
Year ended 30.06.2015		327,744	110,950	107,890	108,904	–

Chapter 5

Fixed assets

Fixed assets are those assets that have a lifespan of more than 12 months; for example, the practice premises, computer equipment, fixtures and fittings, and medical equipment. The surgery property potentially has a longer economic life than equipment and therefore the way that the surgery property is dealt with in the accounts differs from the way that other fixed assets are shown. Fixed assets of a physical nature, such as those just referred to, are also described as tangible fixed assets. An example is shown at the end of this chapter, setting out how fixed assets may appear in the notes to the accounts. Also see the example balance sheet at the end of *Chapter 3*, where the fixed assets are shown in the balance sheet at the top of the page.

Surgery premises

When the surgery premises are owned by the partners in the practice, the surgery property is an asset of the practice and will be included in the fixed asset section of the balance sheet. The value of the premises on the balance sheet may be represented by either the original cost to purchase or to build the property, or the market value of the property. The basis for valuation will be set out in the practice's partnership agreement. The valuation of surgery premises is complex and practices generally engage the services of a specialist valuer to provide a valuation when needed. The premises will need to be valued when there is a change in ownership. This might occur when a partner leaves a practice and sells their share of the property to the remaining partners or to a new partner. It is very important that a specialist valuer is engaged to ensure that a fair valuation for all parties is obtained in what can sometimes be an acrimonious situation.

Some practices require new partners to buy a share of the surgery premises as a condition of becoming a partner. If the value of the property is more than any loan which the practice may have on the property, then the new partner will need to finance their share of this equity by finding cash to invest, typically through obtaining their own additional loan for this amount. This will be an important aspect of their decision whether or not to join the practice. The payment into the practice for property purchase by the new partner would typically be paid out to the group of partners who owned the property previously, because what has happened is that they have sold part of their share of the property to the new partner and this is the money they receive as payment for that sale.

GPs need to get advice from a specialist accountant on tax issues relating to surgery property ownership, which will need to include capital gains tax and stamp duty land tax advice. This particularly applies if a sale of a property, either wholly or a partial share, is being considered.

If partners are not required to buy a share in the surgery premises, then this property may be owned by some of the partners but not all of them. The property would usually still appear as an asset within the practice's fixed assets but a note would be included to acknowledge who owns the property.

If one or more of the property owners is not a partner (typically a retired partner) then the surgery property would no longer be a partnership asset.

In addition, the property might be subject to a valuation exercise at the request of the practice bank manager, who may wish to ensure that the value of the bank's security (the practice property) is still at an appropriate level for the bank's loan requirements. One of the terms of a loan agreement is often that the value of the property should not fall below a certain multiple of the loan. For example, the loan balance should never be more than 75% of the value of the property. If the value of the premises had fallen, this multiple may no longer be achievable and refinancing or, even worse, a repayment of the loan may be required.

In the example at the end of this chapter, the premises are shown at the market value at 1 July 2015, which is £400,000. The mortgage on the property is £250,000, and this figure is shown on the balance sheet (see example at the end of *Chapter 3: Balance sheet*). If this is deducted from the value this gives a net equity value of £150,000. The mortgage amount is a liability and is deducted from the value of the premises to arrive at the net property equity which represents the value of the property, as attributable to the property-owning partners.

Other fixed assets

The value of the other tangible assets (fixtures, fittings, equipment, etc.) in the accounts will be the net book value. This is £1,360 in the example (£400 + £960).

The initial costs of purchasing these assets are not treated as a one-off expense in the profit and loss account. Because the useful economic life of these assets extends for longer than the 12 months of the accounting period, they appear as capital (this can be referred to as 'capitalised on the balance sheet'). However, in the profit and loss account in the year of purchase, and in the accounts for subsequent years, these costs are 'written off' over the agreed period of their economic life. This write-off is called depreciation.

Where an item of equipment is bought costing less than, say, £500, the view would frequently be that this cost could be included as an expense in the profit and loss account rather than including it as an asset. This is because although the piece of equipment had a longer useful life than one year its value was not material to the overall financial wealth of the practice.

It is necessary for the balance sheet to reflect the realistic value of the assets at the accounting year-end. The value of the fixed assets will reduce over time, due to the effect of wear and tear on that asset. The aim in reducing the cost each year by depreciation is to achieve a balance sheet value for the assets equivalent to a reasonable value for those assets at each year-end.

In the example at the end of this chapter, the value of the other tangible assets shown on the balance sheet at 30 June 2016 is £1,360 (computer equipment £400 and office equipment £960). This is known as the net book value. There should always be a note in the accounts that shows how the net book value has been calculated. The note should show the original cost, depreciation and the net book value of the assets.

> **Net book value**
>
> The net book value is the original cost of the asset less the depreciation that has been charged up to the accounts year-end. The net book value is an estimate of the value of the asset if sold at the accounting year-end.

Cost

The note in the accounts relating to net book value of the fixed assets should begin by showing the original cost of the assets, which has been brought forward at the start of the year. This would be the accumulated cost of all assets that the practice has purchased. In this example, the original cost at 1 July 2015 for the computer equipment was £3,000 and for the office equipment £4,000.

During the year ended 30 June 2016 the practice has purchased computer equipment costing £600 and office equipment costing £700 and these figures are added to the cost at 1 July 2015 to arrive at the cost at 30 June 2016 of £3,600 for computer equipment and £4,700 for office equipment.

Depreciation

Depreciation is calculated each year to take account of the wear and tear of the assets. The note shows the depreciation at the start of the accounting period. This is the accumulated depreciation or the total depreciation which has been deducted (charged) in the previous accounting periods. In this example, the accumulated depreciation at 1 July 2015 was £2,000 for computer equipment and £3,500 for office equipment.

The next line is the depreciation charge for the accounting period, which is shown as the 'charge for the year'. Depreciation is calculated using either the straight line method or the reducing balance method (see below for more details). Accountants will recommend what percentage to use to depreciate an asset. In this example the computer equipment is depreciated using a 3 year or 33% straight line method; however, another practice may use 20%. The reason that there is not a set rule on depreciating assets is that it is a matter for judgement what the useful working life of an asset may be. Depreciation is not an allowable expense for tax purposes so variances between depreciation policies do not affect the amount of tax relief available for writing off assets. Instead, capital allowances are claimed and there are rules for these set out in tax legislation (see *Chapter 9: Taxation*).

> **Depreciation charge for year**
>
> The charge for the year is the amount of depreciation which is shown in the profit and loss account as an expense.

Straight line depreciation

In this example, the depreciation charge for the year for computer equipment is calculated based on 3 year straight line. This means that one-third of the cost is classed as depreciation in each year.

The assets held at 1 July 2015 had been written off over the previous two years (cost £3,000, depreciation two-thirds which equals £2,000).

There is one remaining year to write off, giving depreciation on the computer equipment held at 1 July 2015 of £1,000.

The new computer equipment cost £600; this is depreciated by one-third which equals £200.

This gives total depreciation for the year ended 30 June 2016 of £1,200.

This charge for the year figure is added to the accumulated depreciation at 1 July 2015 to give the accumulated depreciation at 30 June 2016 of £3,200.

Reducing balance depreciation

The depreciation charge for the office equipment is 20% reducing balance.

This is calculated by deducting the accumulated depreciation at 1 July 2015 (£3,500) from the cost (including cost of additions in the year to 30 June 2016) at 30 June 2016 (£4,700) and multiplying by 20%, which equals £240 (cost is £4,700 – depreciation of £3,500 = £1,200 × 20% = £240).

The total depreciation charge for the year of £1,440 is shown in the profit and loss account as an expense. Straight line depreciation achieves a faster write-off of assets and is usually used for IT equipment, to acknowledge the likelihood of obsolescence and replacement within a relatively short time frame. The reducing balance method will mean that assets stay on the balance sheet, albeit with a low value for a long time, which is more appropriate for longer-term assets such as desks, filing cabinets, etc.

Net book value

In this example, the original cost of the computer equipment was £3,600, and it has been depreciated by £3,200 to give a net book value at 30 June 2016 of £400. If the practice wanted to sell the computer equipment, this should represent the likely value it would receive for it.

The original cost of the office equipment was £4,700, and it has been depreciated by £3,740 to give a net book value at 30 June 2016 of £960.

The note also shows the net book value at the previous accounting year-end. This is the cost less the accumulated depreciation at the start of the accounting period. In this example, the total cost of the computer equipment and office equipment at 1 July 2015 was £7,000, less the accumulated depreciation at 1 July 2015 of £5,500, giving a net book value of £1,500.

In many partnership agreements the transfer value of equipment will be at the net book value in the accounts, which makes setting a reasonable rate for depreciation important because it establishes the value for the share of assets when a partner is paid out on retirement.

However, historically in a GP practice the balance sheet value of equipment purchased and depreciated has been modest because IT equipment has been provided by the NHS and much funding for other equipment has come from NHS funding or patient donations with no or minimal cost to the practice.

High Street Medical Practice
Notes to the Accounts
Year ended 30 June 2016

20 Fixed assets	Freehold Property	Computer Equipment	Office Equipment	TOTAL
Cost or valuation				
At 1 July 2015	400,000	3,000	4,000	407,000
Additions	–	600	700	1,300
At 30 June 2016	400,000	3,600	4,700	408,300
Depreciation				
At 1 July 2015	–	2,000	3,500	5,500
Charge for the year	–	1,200	240	1,440
At 30 June 2016	–	3,200	3,740	6,940
Net book value				
30 June 2016	400,000	400	960	401,360
30 June 2015	400,000	1,000	500	401,500

Chapter 6

Capital and current accounts

This is the least well understood part of the partnership accounts, but it is extremely important, because it represents the value of the practice and how this is shared between the partners.

The value of the partners' investment in the practice is shown in their capital and/or current accounts in the practice accounts.

The terms 'capital account' and 'current account' can be interchangeable or can be used separately, to distinguish between different types of investment by the partners. The amount in each partner's capital and current account is, in effect, their investment in the practice and would be the cash to which they are entitled should they leave the practice. Whilst they are partners this investment is used to finance the purchase of assets for the practice such as property and fixtures and fittings, and it also provides money in the bank account to meet the day-to-day running costs of the practice.

An example showing the breakdown for a practice's capital and current accounts is shown at the end of this chapter.

Capital accounts

If the partners in a practice own their surgery premises then the cost of the property is included in the accounts. The partners' equity in the surgery property is usually shown separately as a capital account for the partners who own the premises. The net equity of the premises will be the value of the property less the related mortgage. In this example, the net equity in the property is £150,000 (see *Chapter 3: Balance sheet*).

The property may be owned in different shares to the PSRs or, perhaps, not all of the partners will own a share of the property. It is important that the balance sheet clearly shows who owns the property and what their respective shares are.

In this example, only Dr Archie, Dr Bertie and Dr Sidney own the property. Drs Bertie and Sidney own a 25% share each, and Dr Archie owns a 50% share. This ratio is different to the ratio in which they share the profits. Each partner has a capital account to the value of their share of the net equity in the property: Drs Bertie and Sidney's share of the net equity is £37,500 each and Dr Archie's share is £75,000. If the property were to be sold at the balance sheet date, these would be the amounts they would each receive from the sale after the mortgage is repaid. If the property is sold for more than its balance sheet value, the surplus would be divided between the partners in their property sharing ratio and paid to them. Conversely, if the value in the balance sheet proves too high and the property were sold for less than this value, the resulting loss would be divided between the property-owning partners in the property sharing ratio and the payment of their capital accounts to them reduced accordingly.

When there is a change in the value of the net equity in the property (e.g. payments have been made to repay mortgage capital), a transfer is normally made from the partners' current accounts to the capital accounts. This is done to ensure that the capital accounts are always equivalent to the equity in the property. In the example, £20,000 has been paid from the practice bank account to repay the mortgage loan during the year. Effectively the three property-owning partners have taken money out of the practice (from the bank current account) and then paid it back in again (to their mortgage loan account). Looking at the example at the end of this chapter, you can see that Dr Archie's capital account shows a £10,000 transfer in from the current account (increasing the value of his investment in the property), but also a corresponding entry for £10,000 in his current account (reducing the value of his current account). The transaction reflecting the repayment of the mortgage reduces their loan and increases their equity / capital account balances.

If the property is revalued then this is accounted for by increasing or reducing the value of the property on the balance sheet to the revalued amount. Hence, this would increase (or reduce) each partner's capital account. The capital accounts in total would still equal the value of the property, as shown on the balance sheet, less the balance sheet value of the mortgage loan.

Some accountants might recommend that additional capital account funding is held, representing a fixed amount which the practice would require the partners to invest to provide working capital. They might say that the practice needs £50,000 in the bank account, ready to pay bills, whilst waiting for the payment for services which have been delivered. The partners would need to invest their money in the practice to provide this fund. Otherwise cash needs to be left in their current accounts by the partners to provide working capital. Either method achieves the same result, which is to provide working capital funds for the day-to-day management of the practice's cash flow. However, the ultimate decision on appropriate funding levels lies with the partners in the practice. They may prefer the practice to use an overdraft facility to fund the practice's cash flow, assuming that they can negotiate a suitable facility with the practice's bank.

Current accounts

The current account of each individual partner shows their share of profits less drawings.

Drawings

Drawings include the amounts the partners have been paid each month, and also include any taxation and/or superannuation that has been paid by the practice on their behalf.

Current account values are increased by profit earned and decreased by drawings. A partner is entitled to draw their share of profits from the practice, but if their drawings are more than their share of profits, their current account would reduce and possibly go overdrawn. As referred to above, in some practices the partners need to leave some of their profits in their current account each year so that there is cash in the practice bank account to use for working capital. The partners would agree with the accountant each year what might be a reasonable balance to leave in their current accounts.

It is important to appreciate that drawings include not only payments made to each partner each month, but also payments made by the practice on behalf of a partner, such as payments for superannuation, including added years, and taxation. Two partners sharing profits equally may well have different superannuation payments, perhaps due to one partner buying added years, and they will almost certainly have differing income tax liabilities. This would mean in reality that they should take differing amounts of monthly drawings to ensure that, at the end of the year, their respective shares of the wealth in the practice are equal or mirror their relative profit sharing percentages.

In many practices income tax is not paid by the practice. The partners take drawings before tax is calculated and then pay their own tax liabilities. This will often mean that keeping the current accounts in balance from one partner to another is easier to achieve because the calculations are not complicated by the need to factor in the differing tax liabilities of partners. A partner's tax liability encompasses all their income and outgoings, some of which will not be practice based, so tax liabilities are very rarely going to be relative to practice income alone. This can particularly be the case where a partner does extra work on top of their practice work, such as out-of-hours sessions. In such situations, if the practice is paying the partners' tax, then partners with additional income will need to pay part of their tax bill themselves or pay an amount to cover their extra personal tax into the practice each half year when tax payments fall due (31 January and 31 July), so that the practice has funds to cover the personal tax liabilities of each partner.

In addition to it being more straightforward to keep current accounts in balance, paying tax personally rather than through the practice means higher drawings can be paid throughout the year, which can be useful for a partner with an offset mortgage who can use the extra drawings to reduce their house mortgage costs.

The balance on each partner's current account is the money they would be entitled to be paid should they leave the practice. If the balance is shown in brackets (i.e. they had overdrawn) then this amount would need to be repaid to the practice, because it means that the partner has taken more money from the practice than they are entitled to. This may have happened if profits in the year are lower than expected. Profits will not be known until the final accounts have been produced, so the partners' drawings are estimated based on expected profits. If the amount they have drawn is less than the actual profits, the partners may decide to draw out a portion of their available balance. However, they may still need to leave an amount in the practice to meet the day-to-day running expenses, as referred to above.

Current accounts at the start of the year

The note about current accounts in the accounts shows the balance at the start of the accounting period. This is the accumulated amount of money that each partner has not drawn over time. In the example, the current account balances at the start of the accounting period are −£3,000 (i.e. overdrawn) for Dr Archie, £12,000 for Dr Bertie and £8,850 for Dr Sidney. Dr Percy does not have a balance at the start of the accounting period because he only joined as a partner in the accounting period ended 30 June 2016.

Balancing current accounts

It is important that the balances on the current account reflect each partner's commitment to the practice, i.e. their percentage profit share. It is fairly common to see accounts with differing current balances in spite of equal profit shares. For example, partners may share profits in a 50:50 ratio, but one is overdrawn and the other has a high positive balance. This is usually a result of poor financial advice. This situation should not be ignored, because the balances will translate into cash as and when a partner leaves, retires or dies. Furthermore, imbalances can cause animosity between partners, which needs to be avoided for the better working of the practice. Each year partners need to make sure that they understand how their current account has changed in the year and why. This particularly applies where current accounts are not held in the PSR. A specialist medical accountant will look at this as part of the process of presenting the annual accounts to the practice.

In the example, the current accounts at 1 July 2015 were not held in the PSR, which was one-third each at that time. The total for the current accounts was £17,850, which should have been held at £5,950 each. Instead:

- Dr Archie was overdrawn by £3,000, so he was underfunding the practice by £8,950 (£5,950 + £3,000)
- Dr Bertie had a balance of £12,000 so he was overfunding the practice by £6,050 (£12,000 − £5,950)
- Dr Sidney had a balance of £8,850 and so he was overfunding the practice by £2,900 (£8,850 − £5,950).

There are various ways of achieving a balancing position. Deciding how to correct the position will depend on the financial structure of the practice and the financial position of the individual partners.

Where a partner is overdrawn this can easily be rectified if the partner is aware of the situation and has personal funds to pay back into the practice. However, this is rarely the case. The alternative is to give the partner time to correct their balance through reduced drawings over a period of time. This is only possible if the practice cash flow is sufficiently buoyant to be able to accommodate this and also if this approach is acceptable to fellow partners.

Where a partner is not overdrawn but has less than the amount they should have in their current account, the options for correction are similar although, if practice cash flow permits, an alternative is that the other partners may decide to draw down their current accounts so that their balances are brought in line with the lowest balance.

To be fair to all partners a mechanism exists which some practices use to compensate partners with higher levels of investment. Effectively, excess current account balances are a loan to the practice. So the partners with excess current account balances can be paid interest, worked out based on the current account balance at a suitable interest rate. The interest is charged to the practice in the same way as if an external lender, such as a bank, had lent the money.

Overdrawn current account

If a partner's current account is overdrawn this will be shown in brackets. This means that the partner has drawn more money than they are entitled to. This money is owed back to the practice.

In the example, by the time the accounts for the year ended 30 June 2015 were available (which would be the first time that the current account balances at 30 June 2015 were established) the partners were already aware that Dr Percy was joining them in partnership and that the PSR was changing. They therefore agreed to balance to the new PSR of 4:6:8:6. This means that the current account requirement became:

	Ratio	Balances in ratio £	Balances 01.07.15 £	Adjust £	
Dr Archie	4	2,975	(3,000)	(5,975)	Pay in
Dr Bertie	6	4,463	12,000	7,538	Take out
Dr Sidney	8	5,950	8,850	2,900	Take out
Dr Percy	6	4,463	–	(4,463)	Pay in
	24	17,850	17,850	–	

In this case Dr Archie was aware that he had overdrawn and had reserved funds to pay in. This is added to his current account as 'capital introduced'.

Dr Bertie and Dr Sidney were paid the additional amounts and these payments are shown as being deducted from their current accounts as 'capital withdrawn'.

Dr Percy as a new partner has been asked to introduce cash to establish a current account investment in the practice corresponding to his partners. Some practices allow new partners to build up their current account investment by taking drawings which are less than their profit entitlement for an initial period.

Dr Percy could not afford the full £4,463 which he is required to pay in, so the partners agreed that he would pay in £2,000 (which is added to his current account as 'capital introduced') and he will put in the remaining £2,263 by taking reduced drawings over the next 12 months.

Additions to current accounts

Capital (sometimes referred to as 'cash') introduced, as explained in connection with Dr Archie and Dr Percy above, is an addition to current accounts and occurs when there is a need to balance a current account which is overdrawn or provide new or additional current account funding.

Each partner has a share of profits for the year and their profits are added to their current accounts (see *Chapter 4: Profit allocation*).

Each partner pays some expenses which are practice-related from their private bank account, but the expenses are included as an expense in the accounts (see *Chapter 4: Profit allocation*). Effectively the partners have introduced the cash they paid for these expenses into the practice to enable the practice to then claim the expenses as a payment / expense. Therefore the personal expenses claimed are added to the current account in the same way as capital / cash introduced.

Deductions from current accounts

The next part of the current account calculation is the deduction of total drawings from the income available to draw.

Total drawings would include the amounts taken each month for superannuation and taxation (if the practice pays this). For Dr Archie, his monthly drawings for the year totalled £69,811 and the practice had paid superannuation on his behalf of £6,807 for employee contributions and £2,550 for added years.

The property mortgage was repaid by £20,000. The mortgage at 1 July 2015 was £270,000 and this had reduced to £250,000 by 30 June 2016 by virtue of payments made from the practice bank account. Dr Archie's share of the £20,000 repaid is £10,000 because he owns 50% of the property. The £10,000 is classed as a drawing by Dr Archie from his current account.

So, Dr Archie's total drawings for the year were £89,168 (£69,811 + £6,807 + £2,550 + £10,000). This amount is deducted to leave a balance on his current account at 30 June 2016 of £4,160. If Dr Archie left the practice on 30 June 2016, he would be entitled to be paid this amount, which is equivalent to any original or subsequent investment in his current account, plus his profits not yet taken.

The practice needs to establish a drawings calculation policy to ensure, as far as possible, that current accounts are kept in line with the PSR going forward. At its most basic, monthly drawings would be the total cash which the practice considered it could afford to pay out in drawings, which would then be allocated between the partners in their PSR. However, in most practices adjustments need to be made to refine the drawings to match the variances between partners' income and outgoings. The main areas which need to be factored in are:
- seniority
- superannuation variances including added years
- property ownership, where this is not in the PSR
- income tax variances, where applicable
- payment for extra sessions worked.

Seniority

Seniority is paid to the practice quarterly. In our example Dr Archie is entitled to £5,500, Dr Bertie £3,500 and Dr Sidney £1,000 (see example in *Chapter 4: Profit Allocation*). Dr Percy is not entitled to be paid seniority because he became a partner after 31 March 2014, at which point the scheme closed to new entrants (see *Chapter 8: How GPs get paid*). The partners who are entitled to seniority could be paid one-twelfth of their entitlement as part of their monthly drawings. Alternatively, they could be paid quarterly when the seniority is paid into the practice account and this is probably the most common way of paying out seniority to partners. The profit allocation aspects of earning seniority have been covered previously (see *Chapter 4: Profit allocation*).

Superannuation

Superannuation will vary from partner to partner except in the very rare situation where each partner's superannuable income is exactly the same. Even where profits are shared equally this is not likely to apply because each partner's personal expenses are likely to be slightly different from those of other partners.

A more significant disparity can occur where a partner has superannuable income outside the practice; for instance, by virtue of working for another NHS Pension Scheme employer. Because employee superannuation contributions percentages are tiered, the percentage applying to the same practice profits might vary because a GP's external earnings have pushed them up a tier for their superannuation contribution rate. The contribution bands for 2015/16 through to 2018/19 are as follows:

Tier	Pensionable pay	Contribution rate
1	Up to £15,431.99	5.00%
2	£15,432.00 to £21,477.99	5.60%
3	£21,478.00 to £26,823.99	7.10%
4	£26,824.00 to £47,845.99	9.30%
5	£47,846 to £70,630.99	12.50%
6	£70,631.00 to £111,376.99	13.50%
7	£111,377.00 and over	14.50%

Source: NHS Pensions *2015/16 to 2018/19 Tiered Employee Contributions*

Additionally one or more of the partners may be buying added years, or buying additional pension entitlement, through the NHS Pension Scheme (see *Chapter 10: NHS Pension Scheme*) and, where this applies, that partner's drawings need to be reduced to reflect the fact that they are using part of their profits to make this additional pension investment.

In the example, Dr Archie is buying added years and the practice paid £2,550 for him in the year ended 30 June 2016 for this investment. The practice pays the added year contributions because it is deducted (with all GP superannuation contributions) from the monthly GMS/PMS payment to the practice. The total of these monthly payments is shown as a deduction from Dr Archie's current account. Dr Archie's monthly drawings should be reduced by his added years cost, otherwise his drawings would be too high compared to partners who are not buying added years.

Property ownership
Where the surgery property is owned in a different percentage to the PSR, the financial implications of this need to be factored into the drawings calculation (see *Chapter 4: Profit allocation* for information on the profit sharing aspects of this).

In our example, Dr Archie owns 50% of the property and Drs Bertie and Sidney own 25% each. The overall financial implications of the various transactions which feature in the practice accounts relating to property ownership are as follows:

	Property ownership	Notional rent £	Mortgage interest £	Loan repayment £	Net income £
Dr Archie	50%	16,000	(3,738)	(10,000)	2,262
Dr Bertie	25%	8,000	(1,870)	(5,000)	1,130
Dr Sidney	25%	8,000	(1,870)	(5,000)	1,130
	100%	32,000	(7,478)	(20,000)	4,522

Each partner receives their share of notional rent and pays their share of the mortgage interest. This is income and expenses for the property owners and is part of their practice profit (see *Chapter 4: Profit allocation*). From this income they have to repay the capital due on the loan in the accounting year, which totals £20,000. This increases their capital account because they have reduced the mortgage loan, thereby increasing the value of their equity in the property. After they have paid the interest and the capital repayment the property owners still have a profit, referred to as 'net income' in the above table. This can be paid out to them as part of their monthly drawings or as a separate payment.

Payment for extra sessions worked

Such payments would rarely, if ever, be paid as part of monthly drawings because they are by their very nature occasional rather than regular. However, there may be times when a GP is doing regular extra sessions, perhaps as maternity leave cover for a colleague, when it might be appropriate to factor into drawings the value of the extra sessions worked. However, payment would usually be made soon after the session worked as a payment for that session (see *Chapter 4: Profit allocation*).

Establishing appropriate levels for drawings is complex but essential. Where current accounts are not in balance, practices can find themselves in difficult financial discussions between partners, and personal financial situations may become embroiled in practice finances; this can be very destructive to the team relationship. Specialist medical accountants working with GP practices will be able to support the practice through the drawings calculation process to avoid such situations.

High Street Medical Practice
Notes to the Accounts
Year ended 30 June 2016

23 Capital accounts

	Total £	Dr Archie £	Dr Bertie £	Dr Sidney £
Capital account at 1 July 2015	130,000	65,000	32,500	32,500
Revaluation of fixed assets	–	–	–	–
Transfer from current account	20,000	10,000	5,000	5,000
Capital at 30 June 2016	150,000	75,000	37,500	37,500

24 Current accounts

	Total £	Dr Archie £	Dr Bertie £	Dr Sidney £	Dr Percy £
Balance at 1 July 2015	17,850	(3,000)	12,000	8,850	–
Add: Capital introduced	7,975	5,975	–	–	2,000
Allocation of net profit	318,139	87,353	92,663	102,614	35,509
Personal expenses	8,300	3,000	2,000	2,500	800
	352,264	93,328	106,663	113,964	38,309
Less: Monthly drawings	271,345	69,811	78,632	90,152	32,750
Capital withdrawals	10,438	–	7,538	2,900	–
Transfer to capital account	20,000	10,000	5,000	5,000	–
Superannuation – employee	26,871	6,807	7,793	8,912	3,359
Superannuation – added years	2,550	2,550			
Total drawings	331,204	89,168	98,963	106,964	36,109
Balance at 30 June 2016	21,060	4,160	7,700	7,000	2,200

Chapter 7

Specialist medical accounts

The accounts used in this book are prepared by specialist medical accountants. The book has so far covered the main pages that make up a set of accounts:

- profit and loss account
- balance sheet
- profit allocation
- fixed asset note
- capital and current account notes.

This chapter looks at the other pages that may also be included in medical accounts, and describes how this additional information can assist practices in understanding their accounts and using them to help make financial decisions going forward.

Additional / supporting information

The profit and loss account shown in the example at the end of *Chapter 2* shows the income and expenditure of the practice in a summarised format. It is helpful if more information can be provided to aid the process of understanding and using accounts information. Reference is made in the example to numbered notes. The example at the end of this chapter covers those notes. As can be seen by comparing the notes to the profit and loss account, when this information is included in the accounts pack, the GPs in the practice have considerable detail about the figures in their accounts. GPs in a practice should always ask their accountant for any further breakdowns if they are unsure about any figures in the accounts. Such information should be readily available from the accountant's files.

Practice statistics

Accounts prepared by specialist medical accountants are likely to include benchmarking analysis, which provides a practice with information on how it is performing, compared to an 'average practice'. Ratio analysis can be used to highlight to the GPs in a practice where they need to make improvements so that they can increase the profits of the practice. For example, the accountants may look at the practice's level of expenses compared to an average practice, or the levels of income earned compared to an average practice. Ideas for the figures which could be benchmarked are shown below. It is important that benchmark results are considered carefully and discussed with the practice accountant because it is very easy to draw inappropriate conclusions from raw data.

A starting point for consideration might be to look at average patient numbers per GP and compare this to other practices in a benchmark, to consider whether the balance is appropriate from an economic perspective. You need to think about patient needs in your area. High deprivation will mean more GP time is needed, but you will receive income for this through the adjustments for deprivation in your contract pricing.

It is useful to see statistics showing income per patient for the practice's global sum / PMS baseline, QOF, enhanced services and other superannuable and non-superannuable income, and to see this compared to other practices. The comparable data might be from the other practices which your accountant acts for or may be from national data, which would be shown in benchmarks to which your accountant has contributed. Similarly, statistics showing each expense heading, such as medical expenses and staff costs expressed as costs per patient, compared within a benchmark, provide business information for discussion in the practice.

Practice income and expenses can also be expressed as percentages of total income and total expenses and compared within a benchmark.

The dispensing activity can be measured in terms of profit compared to income, again comparing this to other similar practices within a benchmark. Please see *note 11* in the figures below which show the gross profit percentage for dispensing, which could be compared to other practices.

High Street Medical Practice
Notes to the Accounts
Year ended 30 June 2016

2	GMS income	Notes	2016 £	2015 £
	Global sum	3	737,619	725,821
	Directed enhanced services	4	96,647	102,488
	Local enhanced services	5	33,710	34,356
	Quality and Outcomes Framework	6	114,511	112,035
	Support payments	7	14,782	12,678
			995,269	987,378

3	Global sum	2016 £	2015 £
	Global sum	690,365	668,885
	MPIG correction factor	47,254	56,936
		737,619	725,821

4	Directed enhanced services	2016 £	2015 £
	Childhood immunisations	17,921	18,536
	Flu and pneumococcal vaccinations	14,721	15,883
	Extended access	19,378	19,651
	Minor surgery	3,681	5,742
	Learning disability health checks	3,675	4,253
	Dementia	5,614	8,924
	Unplanned admissions	29,657	29,499
		94,647	102,488

5	Local enhanced services	2016 £	2015 £
	Anticoagulant monitoring	9,834	9,756
	IUCD fittings	2,864	3,421
	Near-patient testing	8,673	8,924
	Diabetic clinics	5,486	5,726
	Cardiovascular health checks	6,853	6,529
		33,710	34,356

6	Quality and Outcomes Framework (QOF)	2016 £	2015 £
	Aspiration	78,655	78,412
	Achievement	35,856	33,623
		114,511	112,035

High Street Medical Practice
Notes to the Accounts
Year ended 30 June 2016

7	Support payments	2016 £	2015 £
	Seniority.	10,000	12,678
	Locum cover for sickness	4,782	–
		14,782	12,678

8	Reimbursement of expenses	2016 £	2015 £
	Cost/notional rent	32,450	32,450
	Rates, water charges and clinical waste disposal	14,650	14,350
	Locum reimbursements for attending meetings	3,450	1,750
		50,550	48,550

9	Other NHS income	2016 £	2015 £
	NHS Trust clinical sessions	24,300	24,300
	Training grant	12,400	11,800
		36,700	36,100

10	Other non-NHS income	2016 £	2015 £
	Room rental and service charges	5,500	5,500
	Insurance examinations, reports, etc.	13,780	16,150
		19,280	21,650

11	Dispensing	2016 £	2015 £
	Dispensing fees and on-cost	45,636	42,788
	Cost of dispensed items	32,459	30,980
	Net profit	13,177	11,808
	Percentage return	28.87%	27.60%

12	Medical expenses	2016 £	2015 £
	Medical consumables	7,345	5,345
	Medical protection insurance	15,000	14,650
	Locum cover insurance	2,650	2,550
	Professional subscriptions	3,580	3,450
	Levies	1,460	1,430
		30,035	27,425

High Street Medical Practice
Notes to the Accounts
Year ended 30 June 2016

13	Premises expenses	2016	2015
		£	£
	Rent	450	450
	Business rates	9,950	9,750
	Clinical waste disposal	4,700	4,600
	Light and heat	7,936	10,065
	Buildings and contents insurance	1,575	1,450
	Repairs and maintenance	8,832	15,565
		33,443	41,880

14	Staff costs	2016	2015
		£	£
	Staff salaries	204,960	195,670
	Staff pension contributions	18,575	16,597
	Staff uniforms	620	600
	Staff training and course fees	770	768
	Locum fees	4,580	2,350
		229,505	215,985

15	Administrative expenses	2016	2015
		£	£
	Telephone	5,875	4,567
	Postage, stationery and advertising	4,258	3,569
	Accountancy fees	5,500	5,350
	Professional fees	1,500	350
		17,133	13,836

16	Finance charges	2016	2015
		£	£
	Bank interest and charges	198	158
	Loan interest	7,478	8,476
		7,676	8,634

17	Other expenses	2016	2015
		£	£
	Motor	2,750	1,850
	Sundry expenses	4,229	5,672
	Computer expenses	1,476	1,368
		8,455	8,890

18	Depreciation	2016	2015
		£	£
	Depreciation	1,440	1,550

19	Employers' superannuation	2016	2015
		£	£
	Employers' superannuation	38,000	39,000

Chapter 8

How GPs get paid

GPs provide services *for* the National Health Service, as opposed to being given a contract *of* service, which is the case for hospital doctors. The difference between a 'contract *for* services' and a 'contract *of* service' means that the GP has Independent Contractor status; this gives the GP the right to be self-employed and the right to manage their practice as a separate financial entity. A GP practice is a business, responsible for employing staff and controlling its finances and it is able to choose, to some degree, what services are provided to its patients.

Contracts for services

The core contract for services which a practice will hold will be a General Medical Services (GMS) contract, a Personal Medical Services (PMS) contract or an Alternative Provider Medical Services (APMS) contract. PMS contracts are currently being converted to GMS contracts. NHS England have developed a new model: the multispecialty community provider (MCP) emerging care model.

The GMS contract

The GMS contract is the UK-wide contract between general practices and the relevant government body. In England, from April 2013, this is NHS England (previously called the NHS Commissioning Board). In Wales, Scotland and Northern Ireland contracts are held between the practice and its primary care organisation (PCO).

A GMS contractor can be a sole practitioner GP, a partnership or a limited company. In a partnership, at least one partner must be a medical practitioner. Any partners who are not medical practitioners must be part of the 'NHS family', which means that they must have been an NHS employee or otherwise engaged to deliver services within the NHS. Where a company is used as the contracting vehicle, at least one share must be owned by a medical practitioner. The other shares must be owned by someone in the NHS family.

The GMS contract is for the delivery of primary care services to local communities. The NHS General Medical Services Statement of Financial Entitlement (SFE) sets out the regulations underpinning the GMS contract. The current GMS contract came into effect on 1 April 2004. It is a practice-based contract made up of three main service elements.

- The global sum which covers the main costs of running a general practice and which funds the provision of essential and some additional primary care services.
- The Quality and Outcomes Framework (QOF) which sets standards for achievement in areas of activity (referred to as domains). Payment is based on achieving these standards. Practices can choose whether or not to participate in QOF but it is rare for a practice not to participate.
- Directed enhanced services (DES) which cover additional services that practices can choose to provide.

In addition to the above, other local enhanced services (LES) can be commissioned to meet local healthcare needs.

GMS contract holders are also eligible for reimbursement in certain areas of cost and activity.

The PMS contract

PMS contracts are an alternative to GMS contracts. They are agreed locally and were in existence before the 2004 GMS contract. Many elements of the GMS contract feature in current PMS contracts. These include QOF, enhanced services and seniority. In the past, PCOs have looked to obtain a similar outcome from PMS contracts as from GMS contracts, both in terms of service delivery and costing for those services. This has led to negotiations for PMS contract changes on a practice by practice basis, in particular where the PMS baseline amount – broadly speaking the equivalent of the global sum and Minimum Practice Income Guarantee (MPIG) in a GMS contract – has been priced at a higher level than would be paid for the same services and a similar patient population under a GMS contract in the same PCO area. From April 2014, NHS England commenced negotiations with PMS practices to transfer them to GMS contracts. The pace of this change and the period over which the transition is being achieved varies from area to area.

When a new partner is joining a practice he should ask whether the practice has a GMS or PMS contract. If the practice has a PMS contract he should talk to the practice manager and practice accountant to establish the financial impact of the transition to a GMS contract. Clearly any reduction in the contract value will potentially affect the overall income of the practice.

The APMS contract

This contract is more flexible than a GMS contract, both in terms of services which can be included and the pricing of those services, and also encompasses a wider group of potential contract holders in terms of legal form. APMS contracts are generally of a short duration. In primary care they are typically used as a contractual mechanism for CCGs to engage a provider to step in as a caretaker in a failed practice situation. Alternatively, they might be used to commission specific stand-alone services or groups of services.

Because of the wider group of potential contract holders, GPs working within an APMS contract need to check whether the contract holder is eligible for employer authority status within the NHS Pension Scheme to ensure that their APMS income qualifies as pensionable income in the Scheme.

The MCP contract

This contract is at a developmental stage. The strategy is to build up a model of care to fit the health needs of a specific population. This means that every MCP will be different and will also evolve as needs and solutions are recognised. Vanguards are already working within the MCP model framework, contributing to and informing the development of options for the MCP contract.

This contract is very much about working at scale with the indication that the minimum patient population will be 30,000–50,000. GPs are encouraged to look at working together in larger groupings, either within a GP federation or in a more formal link as part of a super-partnership.

The MCP contract will be for a specific time period; this might be a 10 or 15 year term and will probably include an early break-point. The contract will allow flexibility for variations to be negotiated.

MCP contract holders will need to be a recognised legal entity which would include a limited company or a limited liability partnership (LLP). This will include an appropriately structured GP federation or super-partnership. It could also include a social enterprise arrangement such as a community interest company (CIC).

GPs can be part of an MCP as a partner in a contract-holding LLP or a shareholder in a limited company or CIC holding an MCP contract. Other options would include working on a salaried basis within an MCP contract environment or offering clinical services to the MCP as an independent contractor, maybe as part of a clinical chambers group.

NHS England recognise that moving to the MCP contract environment is a huge step for GPs and indicate that there could be an option for a gradual transition, and also an undertaking that the original GMS contract could be held in a suspended state as a fallback safety net if GPs wanted to step back from the MCP environment. How this might work in practical terms is very difficult to envisage. GPs considering moving to a fully integrated MCP arrangement need specialist accountancy and legal advice, especially on contractual and property issues. GPs participating in an MCP contract as part of a GP federation or super-partnership which retains the underlying features of the GP practice units should find it easier to step back into the GMS environment if appropriate.

Mechanism for making payments to GPs

From April 2013, the Calculating Quality Reporting Service (CQRS) is the system responsible for making payments to GPs. Payments are made by NHS England regional teams. Payments are based on information provided by the General Practice Extraction Service (GPES) which extracts data from GP clinical systems. Payments will continue to be made via the Exeter system, which is an NHS IT system, linking practices to a central database. GPs and their practice managers need to vigilantly check payments to ensure that practices are correctly remunerated for services. The payment system has become increasingly centralised and practices are regularly experiencing errors and delays in payments due to them.

The GMS contract remains the core GP contract and is made up of various key components. Historically the contractual terms were applied UK-wide, but more recently Scotland, Wales and Northern Ireland have developed local variations. The details for the contract components which follow cover the English contract. The framework for the contract terms is set out in the Statement of Financial Entitlements.

Global sum

The global sum is the funding for practices to cover the cost of essential and additional primary care services.

Essential services are:
- management of patients who are ill or believe themselves to be ill with conditions from which recovery is generally expected
- general management of patients who are terminally ill
- management of chronic disease.

Additional services (clawback percentage for non-delivery is shown in brackets) are:
- cervical screening (1.1%)
- contraceptive services (2.4%)
- vaccinations and immunisations (2%)
- childhood vaccinations and immunisations (1%)
- child health surveillance (0.7%)
- maternity services (2.1%)
- minor surgery services (0.6%)
- out-of-hours service (4.92%)

GP practices have a preferential right to provide additional services and normally they would do so, although the majority of practices have opted out of the responsibility for delivering an out-of-hours service. A practice's global sum is reduced for any additional services which are not provided by the percentage attributed to that service (i.e. the percentages quoted above in brackets).

Global sum payments are made to practices according to the needs of their patients and the costs of providing primary care services. The global sum is calculated using the Carr–Hill formula, which is a mechanism whereby the practice list is multiplied by an allocation formula to give a weighted list size. The allocation formula is intended to ensure that the money flows according to patient need. The formula is under review but will not change before April 2018.

> ### Global sum allocation formula
>
> The formula aims to allocate resources to practices based on workload and the unavoidable costs of delivering high quality care to the local population. The allocation formula is based on the following:
>
> - an adjustment for the age and sex of the population of the practice
> - an adjustment for the additional needs of the population, relating to mortality and long-standing illness as attributed to the patient's area of residence
> - an adjustment for list turnover
> - numbers of patients in nursing and residential homes
> - unavoidable costs of delivering the service, e.g. rurality.

An overall weighted list size for the CCG/PCO is generated as the sum of *Practice weighted list sizes* for all practices in the CCG/PCO, and this *weighted list size* is used together with the *weighted population current quarter* to generate the *Practice normalised weighted list size* according to the formula below:

$$\textbf{Practice normalised weighted list size} = \frac{\textit{Practice weighted list size}}{\textit{CCG/PCO weighted list size}} \times \textit{CCG/PCO weighted population}$$

The amount for the global sum is the *Practice normalised weighted list size* multiplied by £85.35 from April 2017 (£80.59 2016/17).

The global sum will also include an amount for Temporary Patients Adjustment (based on 2004 activity levels), superannuation premium and appraisal premium.

The global sum is recalculated quarterly for changes in list size and weighting and is paid monthly.

Minimum Practice Income Guarantee correction factor

The MPIG correction factor was created in 2004 as part of the introduction of the new GMS contract at that time. It was designed to protect a practice's income because 80% of practices would receive less income under the new GMS contract than they did under the old contract.

For those practices that needed an MPIG correction factor, this is an additional monthly payment on top of their global sum. The MPIG correction factor was calculated in 2004, based on the practice's circumstances at the time the new GMS contract was introduced. The MPIG has remained unchanged since 2004, except for some revisions in 2008/09, 2009/10 and 2010/11, when clawbacks were applied as a first stage in removing MPIG from the GMS contract. In the main these clawbacks were modest because they were aligned to GMS pay awards for the years concerned and these awards were minimal.

If a practice started a GMS contract after April 2004 it will have no entitlement to MPIG. If a practice transfers from a PMS contract to a GMS contract then similarly it will have no entitlement to an MPIG, but NHSE may award an MPIG as part of negotiations to transfer to a GMS contract.

GMS practices in England are having their MPIG phased out over seven years, starting from 2014/15, and the funds redistributed between all GP practices within their annual global sum price uplifts. The MPIG is shown in the accounts and practices need to re-evaluate the impact of losing this income in comparison to potential increases in income from other areas of the GMS contract. NHS England produce a ready reckoner in tandem with announcements on contract changes to aid this review process.

Quality and Outcomes Framework

Participation in the Quality and Outcomes Framework (QOF) is voluntary. It is designed to reward high quality care and management through participation in an annual quality improvement cycle. The majority of practices participate fully in the QOF scheme which enables practices to significantly increase their income through QOF achievement.

QOF has a range of national quality standards, based on the best available research-based evidence covering two domains. Each domain contains areas for which there are a number of indicators.

These indicators contain standards (tasks or thresholds) against which the performance of a practice will be assessed and points are then allocated for achievement. Practices are paid for the points awarded using a value which recognises disease prevalence in the practice.

The two English domains are:
- Clinical domain
- Public health.

For 2017/18 there are a maximum of 559 points available to practices across the QOF domains. The points for each domain are as follows:
- Clinical (92 indicators)   435
- Public health (18 indicators)   124
                                      559

Some indicators are subject to certain thresholds (targets).

Practices are paid a monthly aspiration payment and are then entitled to an achievement payment which may be made in one or more instalments at the end of the QOF year (which runs to 31 March annually), when the QOF points achieved can be recognised and evaluated.

The value of a QOF point is £171.20 from April 2017 (£165.18 2016/17). However, because the Contractor Population Index (which provides a population relativity to the calculations) has also increased, the net value of the points for 2017/18 remains as for 2016/17.

Aspiration payments
The monthly aspiration payments are based on either 70% of the practice's achievement for the previous year or a calculation based on the number of points which the practice has agreed with NHS England / the PCO that it is aspiring to in the year.

Achievement payments
Achievement payments are payments based on QOF points achieved for a year. Some points are attributable to completing tasks, as set

out in the QOF performance indicators. Others involve measurement against standards, whereby if the practice does not reach the minimum requirement or only reaches the minimum in a particular indicator then no points are awarded. If the practice achieves between the minimum and maximum scores for that indicator, it is awarded a proportion of the points available. Where a practice reaches the maximum score, it is entitled to full points for that indicator.

The achievement payment is due for payment by 30 June annually.

The value of a practice's clinical and public health domain achievement payments includes factoring in the impact of disease prevalence. This is based on the number of patients on each disease register, known as 'recorded disease prevalence', compared to population averages for each disease. In certain cases, practices can exclude patients. This is known as 'exception reporting'. Strict criteria are used for this process and practices may be required to provide evidence of any patient that is 'exception reported'.

Enhanced services

These are essential or additional services delivered to a higher standard, or services which are not provided and paid for within the GMS global sum.

Enhanced services are split between directed and local. In England from April 2013, NHS England are responsible for commissioning enhanced services, while clinical commissioning groups (CCGs) and local authorities will commission local health services, reflecting their responsibility for local health issues. NHS England will commission directed enhanced services and can still commission local enhanced services, but is unlikely to do so as the local responsibility lies with CCGs and local authorities. GP practices with the right skills will be able to bid for delivery of local health services as part of the CCG and local authority procurement processes.

Directed enhanced services
The following directed enhanced services are commissioned as part of the GMS contract for the 2017/18 contract year:
- childhood immunisations

- influenza and pneumococcal vaccinations
- minor surgery
- violent patients
- Extended Access
- Learning Disability Health Check Scheme.

The Unplanned Admissions DES was withdrawn in April 2017.

Local enhanced services
As the title indicates, these services are commissioned locally by either CCGs or local authorities, reflecting their public health responsibilities. Some of the services which are commissioned are based on national agreed frameworks for service delivery. Practices will be involved with developing and supporting local initiatives which will fall within this framework.

Property reimbursements

GPs are reimbursed for some of their property expenses, including rent and rates reimbursements. The reimbursement is designed to cover the cost of GPs providing accommodation, whether the premises are rented or owned by the GPs. The framework under which reimbursements are made is the Premises Costs Directions.

If a GP practice rents its premises, and the CCG is satisfied with the level of accommodation provided, the CCG will reimburse fully the costs of rent, business rates, water and refuse charges.

Where GPs own their surgery premises they are reimbursed either on a cost rent basis or a notional rent basis:
- cost rent seeks to reimburse the interest charges on the cost of a new or modified surgery; it should be noted that the repayment of capital on any borrowing is for the GP owners
- notional rent is assessed every three years by the District Valuer who determines the current market rent that might reasonably be expected to be paid for the premises. The GP practice can negotiate with the District Valuer to achieve a fair notional rent. The practice should consider whether to instruct an appropriately qualified specialist surveyor to negotiate on their behalf.

GP-owned practices will also be reimbursed for rates, water rates and refuse rates. From 2017/18, practices will also be reimbursed for Business Improvement District levies paid.

The Premises Costs Directions also provide the framework for funding of improvement grants for capital improvement work on practice premises. Where a project is eligible, funding of between 33% and 66% of the cost is available.

Support payments for specific purposes

CQC fees
Practices will receive full reimbursement for CQC fees for 2017/18. Practices will make direct payment to their CQC and then forward their paid invoice to the NHS England regional team for reimbursement.

Indemnity costs
From 2017/18, practices will receive funding on a per-patient basis. This means that this funding will also cover the indemnity costs of any salaried GPs in the practice who should be reimbursed by the practice as appropriate.

Locum costs
NHS England will pay for locums covering maternity, paternity and adoption leave, sick leave and where a GP in the practice has been suspended. The SFE sets out the framework for the costs which are eligible for reimbursement under these arrangements.

Reimbursement for parental leave will be the lower of:
- £1,131.74 for the first 2 weeks and £1,734.18 for weeks 3–20
- the actual invoiced costs in that period.

Reimbursement can pay for external locums and cover provided by GPs who already work in the practice but are not full time.

Practices are also reimbursed for GPs on sick leave. Up until March 2017, the maximum payable was £1,131.74 per week for 26 weeks and then half the amount as agreed with the practice's CCG for the following 26 weeks. From 1 April 2017 the payment becomes an entitlement, removing the discretionary element. Payments will be made after 2 weeks of absence on sick leave. Again, cover can be external locums or from internal GP resource. The amount payable is £1,734.18 per week for 26 weeks and then £867.09 per week for the following 26 weeks.

Prolonged study leave
NHS England may pay an education allowance of £133.68 per week and also pays for locum cover set at a maximum fixed weekly amount of £1,131.74 for GPs taking extended study leave for a pre-approved educational study programme. In practice this reimbursement is rarely utilised by GPs.

Seniority
Seniority payments reward GPs for their working commitment to the NHS. Seniority is only payable to GPs in medical practices and not to employed GPs. The amount a GP receives will depend upon the number of years of reckonable service within the NHS. The number of years of service will be calculated from the date a GP first became registered with the NHS. Entitlement starts after you have been a partner in a GP practice for two years. If you move practices after your two year entitlement period has been achieved then your seniority entitlement follows you to your new practice. However, no new entrants were accepted after 31 March 2014 when the seniority phase-out programme was initiated.

Seniority is also linked to the GP's superannuable earnings. If a GP receives more than the average superannuable earnings, they will receive their full entitlement of seniority. If a GP's superannuable earnings are between one-third and two-thirds of the average, they will receive 60% of their entitlement. If below one-third, the GP will not receive any seniority.

Seniority payments are to be phased out over 6 years starting from April 2014. A target of a 15% reduction has been set for each year. The funding released from this phase-out will be reinvested in the global sum.

The loss of seniority can represent a significant reduction in income for the more senior GPs in a practice.

GP retainer scheme

The purpose of this scheme is to keep doctors who are not working in general practice in touch with general practice. An approved practice is paid a sessional amount when a GP on the scheme works a session in the practice, which funds the practice for providing training and support. The amount payable is £76.92 per session. Additionally, the GP on the scheme is paid a bursary funded by NHS England.

GP Induction and Refresher Scheme

This is not strictly part of the GMS contract, but practices can benefit from this scheme by offering placements to GPs on the scheme who are partially or wholly remunerated by a centrally funded bursary, which is currently £3,500 per month full time equivalent, with additional funding available for indemnity cover and costs of GMC membership and DBS fees. From summer 2017 a pilot scheme called GP Career Plus will be rolled out. The pilot will work with and support about 80 GPs who were considering leaving general practice. It will evaluate measures which may aid retention of experienced GPs in a practice setting.

Dispensing

Some GP practices are authorised or required to provide dispensing services to specific patients. The arrangements for this are not contained in the SFE. They are covered in the 'Dispensing doctors' section (Part 8) of the NHS (Pharmaceutical Services) Regulations 2012. Practices authorised for this are referred to as 'dispensing practices'.

The payments made to dispensing practices for these activities cover the following:

- the basic price of the drug or appliance as stated in the drug tariff, less a discount
- the appropriate dispensing fee; the amount payable is banded, depending on activity levels
- an allowance to cover the VAT payable on the purchase of the product, where the GP practice is not VAT registered (though most dispensing practices are VAT registered)
- any exceptional expenses as listed in the drug tariff.

Certain products are not paid for through this mechanism. Broadly speaking, this relates to certain inoculations which may be centrally supplied as part of the Childhood Immunisation Programme. In addition, the payments do not apply in respect of the supply of oxygen and oxygen therapy equipment, which are covered by separate arrangements with regard to a direct service to the patient.

As referred to above, the payment includes a payment based on the drug tariff, less a discount. If the practice can satisfy its CCG that it is unable to obtain discounts then it may be exempt from the application of the discounts scale. This is only going to apply in rare circumstances, such as where the practice is particularly remote and their suppliers are not prepared to offer discounts for supply. There is also a possibility in such circumstances that the practice could be paid more than the drug tariff if that practice can prove that it has had to buy the drugs at a premium because of its exceptional circumstances.

GP practices which are not authorised to provide dispensing services to patients are entitled to be paid the basic drug price, dispensing fee and VAT for dispensing personally administered items, drugs and also appliances, etc. used for diagnosis. This covers vaccines, anaesthetics and injections, specific diagnostic reagents, IUCDs, pessaries and sutures.

Dispensing service quality scheme
Dispensing practices are eligible for payments under this scheme, provided they meet all of the standards and criteria set for the scheme within agreed timescales. The standards relate to protocols and procedures, staff training, supervision, etc. within the dispensary.

Conclusion on GMS / PMS contract income

So far this chapter has addressed a practice's income from its main NHS practice contract. This contract income is set out in the regulations contained in the SFE and practices (in particular, practice managers) need to make sure that they have a comprehensive understanding of the SFE. This is so that they ensure that a practice does the work necessary to qualify for payment and that it is then paid at the right level for that work and that the payment does actually come through.

Practices receive a detailed monthly statement setting out what has been paid to them and this needs to be carefully checked. In addition, practices are sent further supporting information for payments. An example is the quarterly global sum calculations and these should also be carefully checked. It is useful to show these schedules to the team from time to time so that they have a better understanding of how they are paid for the work that they do; they will then appreciate the importance of recording their clinical work and data they collect during patient consultations, so that this is captured to contribute to the calculations of payments due to the practice.

Other income

Additionally, practices have other activities and sources of income and this is likely to be increasingly the case. Examples of other activities are:

- ad hoc non-NHS work, including private medical examinations for insurance companies, etc., HGV licence medicals, copying file information for Court cases and insurance products, cremation fees
- non-NHS clinical services, such as cosmetic procedures, travel vaccines
- medical officer duties in local community hospitals
- sessional work in district hospitals, as specialists in a field of medicine
- additional specialist clinics within the NHS; for example, outreach clinics providing physiotherapy, occupational therapy and ophthalmology in a local surgery setting, rather than patients travelling to an outpatient clinic in a large district hospital
- attending advisory meetings on health service development or holding posts as board members
- subletting rooms in the surgery premises; practices need to ensure that this income does not exceed 10% of total gross NHS income, otherwise an abatement of the practice's notional rent would be applied (this is unlikely to apply because 10% of gross NHS income in any practice is likely to be a significant figure).

To improve practice income, practices will increasingly need to look to the provision of non-core services either within or outside the NHS. They need to make sure that such services can be delivered profitably without compromising existing income from core services.

Chapter 9

Taxation

Self-assessment was introduced by HMRC from the tax year 1996/97. Each taxpayer is required to complete a detailed tax return, in which they declare all their taxable income and expenditure which is eligible for tax relief. From this information HMRC calculates the individual's tax liability.

Additionally, each partnership is required to complete a partnership tax return, from which each partner takes their own profit share and includes it on their own tax return with details of their own taxable income from other sources.

The nominated partner takes responsibility for completing the partnership tax return and acting as the main contact for the partnership. The partners can choose who to nominate or HMRC will decide for the practice if no one is put forward. All of the partners are jointly liable with their fellow partners for any penalties and interest if the partnership return is late or inaccurate.

Each partner is personally responsible for paying the income tax and Class 4 National Insurance contributions due on their share of the partnership profits.

Calculation of taxable profits

If you are a partner in a partnership, the way that your taxable profits are calculated can be complicated, especially if the practice year-end is not the same as the tax year-end or 31 March year-end. The tax year runs from 6 April to 5 April the following year.

As a partner you are taxed on your share of the partnership profits. The start point for calculation of your share of the taxable practice profits is the profit figure shown on the profit allocation page in the accounts, not on the monthly drawings you have taken out. This is a very common misunderstanding.

Practices do not necessarily prepare accounts to the same year-end date. An individual is taxed on the profits of the accounting period ending in the relevant tax year. For example, accounts prepared to 31 March 2016 will be taxed in the tax year 2015/16 (6 April 2015 to 5 April 2016). For a practice with a June year-end the accounts for the year ended 30 June 2016 will be taxed in the year 2016/17, as this accounting year-end falls into the tax year 2016/17 (6 April 2016 to 5 April 2017).

The figure which appears on the tax return as taxable profits will never be the same as the figure shown in the profit allocation page in the accounts. The reason for this is that some practice expenses are not tax deductible or different claims are made for tax compared to the corresponding claim in the accounts. The main example of this is depreciation, which is replaced by capital allowances as a tax deductible expense.

Capital allowances

Included in the accounts is an expense amount for the costs of depreciating the assets. The rate at which assets are depreciated depends on the assets themselves and the accountant's professional view on the appropriate depreciation rate (see *Chapter 5: Fixed assets*). Depreciation is not an allowable expense for tax purposes and so it is replaced by capital allowances.

Capital allowances are complex. This section aims to provide an explanation of how the main rules will affect a practice and its partners most of the time, rather than providing a comprehensive coverage of this topic.

The main capital allowances are the annual investment allowance (AIA), first year allowance (FYA) and writing-down allowance (WDA).

Annual investment allowance

The AIA applies to most new purchases of plant and machinery (not cars) in the accounts year. From 1 January 2016 the rate has been a 100% allowance on total purchases up to £200,000 per annum. From 1 April 2014 to 31 December 2015, the 100% allowance was available on total purchases up to £500,000 per annum.

Plant and machinery includes IT and office equipment and furnishings. Therefore in the typical GP practice annual scenario, the AIA is available as a 100% write-off on most possible equipment purchases in an accounting year.

First year allowance

A 100% FYA is available for expenditure on certain specific types of asset. The assets that qualify for FYA are:
- new cars with CO_2 emissions of not more than 75 grams per kilometre (g/km)
- certain designated energy-efficient equipment
- certain environmentally beneficial (currently water-efficient) equipment
- equipment for refuelling vehicles with natural gas, biogas or hydrogen fuel
- new zero-emission goods vehicles, such as electric vans.

Where a practice builds new surgery premises it is likely that there are integral features within the building which will qualify for FYA under the energy and environmental categories. You should involve a specialist in this area during the build phase to consider the materials and equipment used to ensure that you maximise your FYA claim which can be significant and, therefore, very advantageous in the initial working life of a new build project.

FYA can also be referred to as enhanced capital allowances.

Writing-down allowance

Writing-down allowances are annual allowances that reduce, or 'write down' any balance of capital expenditure on plant and machinery for which you have not been able to claim either the AIA or FYA, and also any residual balances of expenditure that you have brought forward from the previous accounting period.

There are two rates of WDAs for plant and machinery. To calculate them, you first group your expenditure into different pools.

- **Main pool** which covers expenditure on most items, including vehicles (those which are 100% business use) with CO_2 emissions not exceeding 130 g/km. The current WDA rate is 18% per annum.
- **Special rate pool** covers special rate expenditure including long-life assets, integral features, certain thermal insulation and cars (those with 100% business use) with CO_2 emissions exceeding 130 g/km. The current WDA rate is 8% per annum.

WDA for expenditure on short-life assets, or assets that you have used partly for non-business purposes, are calculated individually for each asset concerned. This will apply to the partners' cars which typically would have some non-business use. That expenditure is therefore included in a separate pool for each asset, known as a single asset pool. A partnership will have several single asset pools, one for each partner's car and, if relevant, one for short-life assets.

Short-life assets are those assets with a likely useful life of less than eight years. In reality the cost of such assets is usually written off for tax by the AIA so it is only if a practice buys assets which exceed the AIA in an accounts year that you would need to consider the separate pool for short-life assets.

The rate of WDA to apply to each of these separate pools will depend on the type of asset on which the expenditure was incurred. In GP practices this will in all probability only apply to the partners' cars.

Capital allowances on cars bought on or after 6 April 2009

The capital allowances you can claim on your cars are based on CO_2 emissions, which are shown on the car's V5 certificate.

- Where CO_2 emissions are over 130 g/km the WDA is currently 8% per annum.
- Where CO_2 emissions are 130 g/km or less but more than 75 g/km the WDA is currently 18% per annum.
- Where CO_2 emissions are 75 g/km or less, FYA is available and you can claim up to 100% allowance in the accounting period of purchase.

The percentages referred to above are the percentages claimed before reducing your claim to account for non-business use. If you buy a car with CO_2 emissions between 75 and 130 g/km and you use your car 40% for practice use, then your 18% claim is reduced by 60% to arrive at your tax claim. Here is an example covering more than one year for a car with CO_2 emissions between 75 and 130 g/km, costing £20,000. The car is sold in year 4 for £15,000.

		Pool	Private use	Private use	Tax allowance	Tax charge
		£	%	£	£	£
Cost		20,000				
WDA year 1	18%	(3,600)	60%	(2,160)	(1,440)	
Carry forward at end of year		16,400				
WDA year 2	18%	(2,952)	60%	(1,771)	(1,181)	
Carry forward at end of year		13,448				
WDA year 3	18%	(2,421)	60%	(1,452)	(968)	
Carry forward at end of year		11,027				
Part exchange value on sale in year 4		15,000				
Balancing charge (profit)		3,973	60%	2,384		1,589

Each year the original cost is reduced by the WDA claim (before it is adjusted for private use). The 18% claim for the next year is then applied to the carry forward value at the end of the previous year. When the car is sold the sale value is compared to the tax value at the end of the previous accounting year. If it is more, a profit (charge) has been made and this is taxable income, after the private use adjustment. If it is less, there is a loss (allowance) and a tax claim can be made, again after the private use adjustment.

Personal expenses

Self-employed GPs can claim their expenses, which are 'wholly and exclusively' incurred in the performance of their duties. The following expenses can be claimed for tax relief:

- motor expenses (business use only)
- professional subscriptions
- telephones (including mobiles) – business use only
- professional proportion of use of home, effectively a study allowance
- personally bought drugs and instruments
- printing, postage and stationery
- medical books and journals
- course fees
- personal accountancy fees.

Personal expenses will generally be paid from the partner's personal bank account and, therefore, each GP is responsible for recording and collating their expense claims each year. Many specialist medical accountants will supply their clients with a template spreadsheet to use to record the transactions through the year and provide a year-end summary. GPs must keep supporting invoices for payments made, in case the practice has an HMRC enquiry. These records must be kept for six years. They should also keep a mileage log documenting all journeys made, to support their claim for the business use of their car.

For an employed GP, the expenses that can be claimed have to be 'wholly, exclusively and necessarily' incurred in the performance of their duties. The additional criterion of 'necessity' makes a significant difference between the expenses of a self-employed GP and those of an employed GP. Employed GPs would generally only be able to claim the following:

- professional subscriptions
- business mileage using the HMRC rates.

Some GPs may have partnership income, separate self-employed income (for instance from working sessions for an out-of-hours organisation) and employment income from working sessions in a hospital unit.

A reasonable attempt needs to be made to make separate expense claims for each activity.

How self-employed GPs pay their tax

Income tax calculation

Personal allowance

The personal allowance is a tax-free amount available to all potential tax payers. You can earn up to the personal allowance and not pay any tax on your income. The personal allowance for 2017/18 is £11,500 (the 2016/17 allowance was £11,000). The allowance is deducted from income before the tax rates illustrated below are applied to work out your tax liability.

However, there is a restriction applied to the personal allowance which potentially affects GPs. Where a GP's taxable income exceeds £100,000, the personal allowance is reduced by £1 for every £2 of income above that £100,000 limit. This reduction applies irrespective of age. As the personal allowance in 2017/18 is £11,500 this means that when taxable income exceeds £123,000 (£100,000 plus (£11,500 × 2)) no personal allowance is available. It also means that the extra income between £100,000 and £123,000 has an effective tax rate of 60%. The following example demonstrates this.

Scenario A		Scenario B	
	£		£
Taxable income	100,000	Taxable income	112,000
Personal allowance	(11,500)	Personal allowance**	(5,500)
Income on which tax is payable	88,500	Income on which tax is payable	106,500
Tax payable:		Tax payable:	
£33,500 × 20%	6,700	£33,500 × 20%	6,700
(£88,500 − 33,500) × 40%	22,000	(£106,500 − 33,500) × 40%	29,200
	28,700		35,900
**Personal allowance is £11,500 − ((£112,000 − £100,000) / 2)			

The income in Scenario B is £12,000 (£112,000 − £100,000) more than in Scenario A. The tax payable in Scenario B is £7,200 (£35,900 − £28,700) more than in Scenario A. £7,200 as a percentage of £12,000 is 60%.

Many GPs, when looking at the profit allocated to them in the accounts, become concerned that they may be affected by the personal allowance restriction. However, the figure for a GP's profit in the practice accounts is not the same as a GP's personal taxable profit figure. For instance, the accounts profit will be before deduction for the tax relief available on superannuation contributions paid in the year. The personal allowance restriction is based on taxable income and this will be practice taxable profits after deduction of employee, employer and (if applicable) added years superannuation payment in the tax year.

If a GP is doing other work, such as out-of-hours sessions, or has significant other income, such as rental income, then this would also be included in the taxable profit figure and this might lead to a full or partial restriction of the personal allowance.

What can you do if you find yourself in this position?
- You could reduce your practice income by reducing your sessions or paying a locum to cover some of your work and paying for the locum yourself. Your partners would need to be agreeable to this.

- You could reduce any other earned income by stopping or reducing the extra work which you do.
- You could consider using a limited company for this income; this option is considered later in this chapter.
- If your other income takes you over £100,000, you could transfer certain income, e.g. rental income, by transferring the underlying asset to your spouse / civil partner and your income would be reduced accordingly. Obviously this needs to be the right course of action in other ways, not just for tax purposes.
- You could reduce your taxable income to £100,000 by paying into a personal pension or self-invested pension plan or by making gift aid payments. Whilst this might free up your personal allowance and reduce your tax liability, it does require a pension or gift aid payment to achieve this and therefore affordability needs to be considered. However, a personal pension payment against income in the £100,000 to £123,000 band would effectively attract 60% tax relief.

If your income is significantly over the upper limit of the restriction, which in 2017/18 is £123,000, then you may accept that the £23,000 band of income suffers a 60% tax rate. From £123,000 up to £150,000 the tax rate reverts to 40%. If your income is significantly above £123,000 then you may not wish to reduce your income to £100,000 or less as this would be a significant reduction in your income and may not be affordable.

In some circumstances you may be eligible for a married couple's allowance, or a marriage or blind person's allowance.

Tax rates

Under self-assessment, individuals pay tax at the end of January and July each year on any income which has not been taxed at source. Depending on their tax bands they will also pay tax at the higher tax rate of 40% or 45% on any income which has suffered tax deduction at source at the 20% rate. UK dividend income is taxed at different tax rates to other types of income. For 2017/18, the first £5,000 of dividend income is tax-free. Above this the tax rate is 7.5% if your total taxable income for 2017/18 is below £33,500, or 32.5% for taxable income between £33,501 and £150,000, or 38.1% for taxable income over £150,000.

From 2016/17 a new regime for taxing savings income was introduced. Savings income includes interest from bank and building society accounts, interest from credit unions and National Savings, interest distributions (but not dividend distributions) from authorised unit trusts, open-ended investment companies and investment trusts, income from government and company bonds, income arising under the accrued income scheme, chargeable life assurance gains and most types of purchased life annuity payments.

The starting tax rate for savings income is 0% and this is available on the first £5,000 of savings income. However, the starting rate is not available where the taxpayer has any taxable income in excess of £5,000 other than the income from savings or life assurance gains, employment termination payments or dividends. Additionally a taxpayer may be eligible for a personal savings allowance on savings income. GPs are generally not eligible for the starting tax rate for savings income because their overall taxable income usually exceeds £5,000. However, if their taxable income overall is between £0 and £43,000, they would be eligible for a personal savings allowance on savings income up to £1,000 or £500 where taxable income overall is between £43,000 and £150,000.

The table below shows income tax bands and rates.

In allocating income to tax bands, non-savings income is taxed first, then savings income and finally dividends. Non-savings income includes income from employment, profits from self-employment, pensions, income from property and taxable benefits. These calculations are complicated and your accountant will use specialist tax software to work this out for you.

2016/17			2017/18	
Band	Rate		Band	Rate
£	%		£	%
0–32,000	20*		0–33,500	20*
32,001–150,000	40**		33,501–150,000	40**
over 150,000	45***		over 150,000	45***

* Except dividends which are taxed at the 7.5% rate where they fall within this tax band.

** Except dividends which are taxed at 32.5%.

*** Except dividends which are taxed at 38.1%.

National Insurance contributions calculation

Self-employed GPs are required to pay both Class 2 and Class 4 National Insurance contributions (NICs). Class 2 is currently £2.85 per week (in the tax year 2016/17 it was £2.80 per week) which is paid with your half-yearly income tax payments. Class 4 is calculated based on a GP's taxable profits.

The following table shows Class 4 NIC bands and rates.

2016/17			2017/18	
Band	Rate		Band	Rate
£	%		£	%
0–8,060	0		0–8,164	0
8,061-43,000	9		8,165-45,000	9
over 43,000	2		over 45,000	2

Class 4 NIC is calculated and paid with income tax liabilities on 31 January and 31 July.

As can be seen, Class 4 NIC makes a significant impact on half-yearly payments to HMRC. It is effectively an additional tax charge and should not be overlooked in considering tax liabilities.

How income tax and Class 4 NICs are paid to HMRC

The due dates for payments are 31 January and 31 July each year.

On each date a payment on account for a tax year is paid. On 31 January this is a payment on account for the year in which that payment falls. For instance, the first payment on account for the tax year 2016/17 is made on 31 January 2016. The second payment on account is made on 31 July 2016. The payment on account is usually half of the previous year's total tax liability (see example below). Once your tax return has been prepared you may have to make a balancing payment or you may be due a refund, depending on whether your actual tax liability for the year is more or less than the payments on account which you have already made. This is paid on 31 January following the end of the tax year, with the payment on account for the

Example of tax payments for 2016/17

31 January 2017
First payment on account 2016/17   £15,000

(There may also have been a balancing payment due to be made for 2015/16 on 31 January 2017.)

31 July 2017
Second payment on account 2016/17   £15,000

Once the 2016/17 tax return has been completed the actual tax due will be compared with the payments on account and any difference will be paid on 31 January 2018. For example, if the total tax due for 2016/17 was £34,000 then the tax liability in January 2018 would be:

31 January 2018
Balance 2016/17 (£34,000 − £15,000 − £15,000)	£4,000
First payment on account 2017/18 (half of the tax due 2016/17)	£17,000
Total tax payable	£21,000

31 July 2018
Second payment on account 2017/18	£17,000

next tax year. So if your income has gone up since the previous tax year, you will have a balance due in the following January together with the first payment on account for the following tax year.

If practice profits go down, you will have overpaid tax through your payments on account and this overpayment will be repaid by HMRC as soon as your tax return has been processed. In this situation it may be possible to anticipate this overpayment and reduce your payments on account. For example, if your accounts were complete before the 31 July payment so you knew that you owed less tax, you could apply to pay a correspondingly lower payment on account.

Joining and leaving a practice

When a new partner joins a practice they must notify HMRC by completing form SA401. They will then need to seek advice from their accountant or the practice accountant on their likely future tax liabilities so that they can understand how they fit into the tax system and how much they need to be saving for tax if they are paying their own tax. This is complex and depends on a number of factors:

- Has the GP been employed, self-employed or not working at all before joining the practice?
- Will they work full-time in the practice or will they work part-time and continue to have other earnings / income?
- What is the practice year-end date in relation to the date the partner joined the practice and also in relation to the tax year?

A specialist medical accountant will be able to work through scenarios with GPs on an individual basis and give advice as necessary. The recommendation is to ask for this advice as soon as you join a practice. As your profit share builds up, it can take several years before you are on regular half-yearly tax payments so you will need to get advice to help you properly plan for your tax payments.

Similarly, when leaving a practice either to retire or to move to another job or practice, a GP should seek advice from the practice accountant or their own accountant to make sure that they are forewarned of future potential tax liabilities.

Where a practice has a year-end which is not 31 March or 5 April, i.e. is not in tandem with the tax year, GPs joining and leaving the practice will have a more complex initial and final taxable profit calculation, involving overlap profits. This is a complex issue and best addressed by obtaining advice for individual circumstances from a specialist medical accountant.

Using a limited company

A limited company pays corporation tax, as opposed to the income tax and Class 2 and 4 NICs which a GP pays on their income. The corporation tax rate for companies is 19% in 2017/18. It was 20% for 2016/17. Therefore this might appear to be an attractive vehicle to use, potentially enabling a GP to save tax. However, there are many reasons why this will not necessarily achieve a tax saving or might not be practical or possible.

Whilst a company may pay 19% tax, for a GP to be able to take income out of the company this would be either as a salary with income tax and Class 1 NICs payable (which could well involve a higher NIC charge than through the self-employed route) or as dividends. These, as can be seen above, attract a further tax charge where a taxpayer's dividend income exceeds their £5,000 dividend tax allowance (for 2017/18), but no NIC, because NICs are only payable on earned income.

A limited company with the dividend income extraction route would probably be more tax efficient than the self-employed route, especially if it were reasonable for a lower earning spouse / civil partner to be a shareholder in the company with the GP and receive their dividends if a lower tax rate applies.

However, if the income in the company was superannuable, the GP's employee and added years (if applicable) superannuation contributions would not attract tax relief. This is because you have to have taxable earned income to set this pension cost against and dividends are investment income, not earned income. The company would get tax relief against company profits for the employer's superannuation contributions only. This reduced tax relief on superannuation contributions will significantly dilute the potential tax efficiency of using a limited company and the structure may well not be tax efficient at all. For the income to be superannuable, the limited company would need to be the holder of an NHS contract and be registered with the NHS Pension Scheme as a Scheme employer. This is likely to apply to a GP practice and for this reason very few GP practices have found it tax efficient to operate as a limited company.

If the income in the company was not superannuable (because the company was not a registered NHS Pension Scheme employer) tax relief on the superannuation would not be an issue. It is possible that in transferring work to a limited company you were converting income which, if you earned it yourself, was superannuable, into income which was not superannuable (because it was passing through a company). This might not achieve the appropriate outcome for you in terms of your plans for your pension funding. On the other hand, you might wish to reduce your superannuation payments for other reasons, such as planning around the Annual Allowance and/or Lifetime Allowance; a limited company might then be a good route for you (see *Chapter 10: NHS Pension Scheme*).

This is a complex area and GPs need to obtain specialist tax and investment advice to consider their individual circumstances.

Tax payments in the practice accounts

Tax payments may not feature in the practice accounts at all. If tax is paid by the individual GPs from their personal bank accounts then no tax payments will be made from the practice bank account and, therefore, there will be no tax figures in the practice accounts.

If the practice pays the partners' tax liabilities, the payments will be analysed to the partner to whom the tax payment relates, and the total paid in a year will be a deduction from that partner's current account, in the same way that drawings are a deduction (see *Chapter 6: Capital and current accounts*).

There are situations where the practice may pay tax for a GP because during part of their working week they are employed and they are doing that work in practice time, thus making the employment income practice income. Because it is an employment, the GP doing this work will be an employee of whatever body commissions this work and income tax, NIC and superannuation, as applicable, will be deducted from the salary before the payment of the net income is made to the practice. In this situation the practice has effectively paid the income tax, NIC and superannuation on behalf of the GP and these payments will also be a deduction from the GP's current account.

Because the income is shared between the partners it may seem unfair that the one GP has suffered the whole of the income tax, NIC and superannuation on this income, not just on his equivalent profit share. Therefore this needs to be adjusted for in the practice tax calculations to arrive at a fair position between the partners. This is done by adjusting the profit share, as demonstrated in this example.

	Total £	Dr Archie £	Dr Bertie £	Dr Sidney £
Taxable profits split in PSR	285,000	95,000	95,000	95,000
Salaried income earned by Dr Sidney	(25,000)			(25,000)
Taxable profits from self-employment	260,000	95,000	95,000	70,000
Taxable profits from employment				25,000
Total taxable profits from practice		95,000	95,000	95,000

Dr Sidney will pay self-assessment tax on £70,000, whereas Drs Archie and Bertie will pay self-assessment tax on £95,000 each. In this way Dr Sidney will pay less tax on self-assessment income than his partners despite having the same profit share in the practice, because he has already separately paid tax on the £25,000 of his profit share which is employment income.

This adjustment will also flow through so that he pays less superannuation for the same reason. In fact an inequality will occur in respect of superannuation because as an employee Dr Sidney's employer's superannuation is paid by his employer, whereas the employer's superannuation on practice profits has to be paid by the GP partners. Where such a benefit is material, a profit share adjustment might be considered to arrive at a fairer position between the partners.

Dr Sidney may pay more NIC than his colleagues because he is paying Class 1 NIC on the salary. He may also overpay NIC by paying Classes 1, 2 and 4; the practice accountant will need to consider whether a claim for repayment of overpaid NIC should be made.

Chapter 10

NHS Pension Scheme

Understanding how the NHS Pension Scheme works is very important for GPs. The Scheme offers the opportunity to build up an entitlement to a substantial pension. However, the contribution costs have increased in recent years and the taxation of pensions has become more complex. This chapter gives a brief introduction to the Scheme and to the taxation issues of which a GP needs to be aware.

GPs holding GMS, PMS or APMS contracts, or operating as self-employed locums, are 'practitioner' members of the NHS Pension Scheme. At present there is a lack of clarity as to whether GPs working within an MCP contract will be able to pension their income through the Scheme. NHS England are negotiating on this. There is also an 'officer' section of the Scheme of which employees of the NHS are members. GPs automatically become members of the Scheme when they start their first post in the NHS. This could be in the officer Scheme in an employed job or in the practitioner Scheme in a practice or as a self-employed locum. GPs can decide not to join the Scheme but this is very rare at the start of a GP's career. Generally GPs would join the Scheme at the outset of their NHS career.

There are different sections of the Scheme which apply depending on when you join the Scheme and your age. There have been opportunities to migrate from older versions of the Scheme to more recent versions.

The oldest section of the Scheme is the 1995 section. If you joined the NHS Pension Scheme before 1 April 2008 then you joined the 1995 section. The 2008 section was introduced for new members from 1 April 2008. 1995 section members were given the opportunity to move to the 2008 section. Very few chose to do so because the normal retirement age for the 1995 section is 60 and for the 2008 section it is 65.

From 1 April 2015 a new section, the 2015 section, was introduced. All scheme members who were aged 50 or older on 1 April 2012 remain in their original section, i.e. 1995 or 2008. If your date of birth is 2 September 1965 or later, you moved to the 2015 section on 1 April 2015. For members with dates of birth between 1 April 1962 and 1 September 1965, you will move to the 2015 section on a tapered basis depending on your exact date of birth.

The normal retirement age for the 2015 section is your state pension age. All sections of the Scheme offer retirement options before the section's normal retirement age, but pensions taken earlier are actuarially reduced.

For those members who are now in the 2015 section, but have earlier 1995 or 2008 membership, then their pension entitlement which has built up in the earlier sections stays in that section with the rules for retirement and other benefits following the specific section's rules. This means that there are currently many Scheme members who can take part of their pension, at its full rate, at age 60, from their 1995 section pot and the rest of their pension entitlement at full rate at state pension age from their 2015 pot.

Pension entitlement is based on earnings and contributions to the Scheme are similarly based on annual income levels. Contributions to the NHS Pension Scheme are often referred to as superannuation payments.

A GP's pension contributions are calculated based on their NHS profits. These profits are based on the practice accounts and partnership self-assessment tax return. The practice profits are adjusted to take out any non-NHS income and its related expenditure to arrive at the profit attributable to NHS activity. GPs are required to complete and sign an annual form detailing the calculation of their NHS profits. This is called an 'annual certificate of pensionable profit' and has to be submitted by 28 February annually, covering income for accounts years falling in the previous NHS year to 31 March. The certificate for accounts years ending in the year ended 31 March 2017 will need to be submitted by 28 February 2018. Where a GP in a practice has other NHS income, earned outside the practice environment, then this income will also need to be declared annually.

Employee and employer contributions

GPs pay employee and employer contributions. The employer contribution is 14.3% of NHS profits. The reason that a GP pays their own employer's superannuation is that their employer (the NHS) is deemed to have paid to the practice, within the GMS global sum or PMS contract sum, funding for employer superannuation, so the subsequent payment of employer contributions by a practice for a GP is the payment of this funding across to the Scheme.

The level of employee contributions depends on a GP's NHS income because the contributions are tiered.

Tier	Pensionable pay	Contribution rate
1	Up to £15,431.99	5.00%
2	£15,432.00 to £21,477.99	5.60%
3	£21,478.00 to £26,823.99	7.10%
4	£26,824.00 to £47,845.99	9.30%
5	£47,846 to £70,630.99	12.50%
6	£70,631.00 to £111,376.99	13.50%
7	£111,377.00 and over	14.50%

Source: NHS Pensions *2015/16 to 2018/19 Tiered Employee Contributions*

Tiered contributions can mean that partners in a practice who all earn the same level of practice income may pay different levels of employee superannuation contributions on that practice income if they do other NHS work, because that other income may take them into a different band for contributions.

Added years contributions

A GP can also buy additional NHS pension benefits. Up until 31 March 2008 a GP could take out a contract with the Scheme to buy added years. They paid extra to their NHS Pension pot, based on a fixed percentage, which was actuarially evaluated by the Scheme administrators at the outset of the added years contract. Where a GP has transferred to the 2015 section of the Scheme, added years still attach to their 1995 section pension entitlement.

Purchase of additional pension entitlement

Since 1 April 2008 members have had the option to buy an additional NHS pension of up to £5,000 per annum. Purchases can be made in blocks of £250 and the additional pension will be claimed at normal pension age. The cost of buying this additional benefit is fixed at the time of purchase and can be spread over 20 years or the period to retirement, if less, or be paid for by a lump sum investment at the outset. The benefits can be based on the GP's life expectancy or can be enhanced to also provide a spouse's additional pension, subject to an increased cost to purchase.

Superannuation payments in the practice accounts

Superannuation is paid by the practice for its GPs. Each month when the global sum or baseline contract payment is made to the practice, superannuation is deducted from the amount due. The monthly GMS/PMS statement shows the breakdown of the superannuation deductions so that these can be analysed to each GP and included in the accounts as a deduction against each GP's current account. These monthly payments on account are provisional, based on estimates established at the start of April each year.

When the year-end superannuation certificates are processed there will usually be a balancing payment or repayment which will normally be paid / repaid to the practice in March each year. These figures will be included in the total deducted from each GP's current account.

Because the balancing payment / repayment is paid in arrears, accountants will seek to estimate the balance due so that a debtor or creditor can be included in the accounts. In this way a GP's current account at a year-end date will more closely represent what would be due to them if they left the practice at that time. If the debtor or creditor wasn't included because any balance of superannuation is paid through the practice's GMS/PMS payments mechanism, even where a partner has since left the practice, then this would need to be separately paid to, or recouped from, the retiring partner at a later date. As this can sometimes be difficult to achieve, particularly if there has been an acrimonious departure, ensuring that the adjustment is recognised in the accounts and deducted from a partner's current account at the appropriate time protects all parties.

Tax relief on superannuation contributions

GPs are eligible for tax relief on the superannuation payments which are physically made in a tax year. This is claimed on the individual GP's self-assessment tax return each year. The figure to be included in the tax return is the total of the actual payments in the actual tax year. Where debtors or creditors are included in accounts, as mentioned above, these have to be excluded when working out the superannuation figure for tax returns.

The Annual Allowance is a measure which establishes whether your pension benefits (in the case of a defined benefit pension scheme such as the NHS Scheme) have grown over a permitted level. In the case of a defined contribution scheme or a personal pension plan the measure is the actual contributions paid in the year. Prior to 6 April 2011 the

Annual Allowance was £255,000 per annum but this was reduced to £50,000 per annum from 6 April 2011, and £40,000 per annum from 6 April 2014. From 6 April 2016 this can be reduced to £10,000 for higher earning GPs. This is likely to mean that higher-earning GPs, particularly those nearer retirement age, or GPs with unusual earnings growth in a tax year, may now exceed the Annual Allowance. If a GP exceeds the Annual Allowance, a tax charge at their top rate of tax is applied to the excess. Effectively a GP would no longer be receiving full tax relief on their superannuation contributions.

Reviewing a GP's annual allowance position has become increasingly complex as the tax legislation in this area has developed. Advice from a specialist medical accountant and an independent financial advisor with sector specialist knowledge should be sought.

The Lifetime Allowance sets a level above which your pension will be subject to a Lifetime Allowance tax charge at retirement. The level is reducing; it is currently £1m.

The rule of thumb Lifetime Allowance valuation is your NHS pension multiplied by 23. This means that GPs expecting a pension of more than £43,478 per annum (£1m divided by 23) will potentially exceed the Allowance and suffer an additional tax charge of 25% on the slice of their pension above the Allowance, and 55% on their lump sum above the Allowance. In addition, any non-NHS pensions need to be valued and brought into the calculation.

The above is a very brief description of what is a very complex issue. There are tax planning steps which can be considered to mitigate the likely outcome. Specialist independent financial advice should be sought if you are likely to be affected by this.

Other pension funding

A GP may wish to make pension contributions outside the NHS Scheme and this is an option they can consider with appropriate investment advice. There is a facility to make additional voluntary contributions through the NHS Scheme or payments can be made into other investment-based pension schemes, such as personal pension plans or self-invested personal pensions. However, GPs need to monitor their position, particularly with regard to the Annual Allowance and Lifetime Allowance referred to above, because a GP's total pension funding is measured when considering whether these allowances have been exceeded.

Glossary

Assets
Assets are items that the practice owns or amounts that are owed to
it. For example, if it owns the premises, this is an asset. Any money in
the bank account is also an asset. The assets can be divided into 'fixed'
and 'current' assets. Fixed assets represent long-term assets (often the
premises), whereas current assets represent short-term assets such as
cash.

Balance sheet
The balance sheet shows the values of the assets and liabilities on a
single day. In contrast, the profit and loss account shows the income
and expenses for the accounting period and usually covers a 12-month
period.

Capital and current accounts
The terms 'capital account' and 'current account' describe the partners'
share of the wealth in the practice. The total of a partner's capital and
current account is the amount of money they have invested in the
practice and it will be this amount that they are entitled to when they
leave.

Creditors and accruals
These are the amounts owed by the practice to third parties at the year-end. They might include, for example, the cost of drugs purchased during the accounting period, but not paid for by the time of the year-end.

Current assets
Current assets are short-term assets which can be turned into cash within the next 12 months. These include stock of drugs, debtors and bank funds. The value of these will change from day to day. For example, the money in the bank account will change due to income being received and overheads being paid.

Debtors
Debtors comprise money that is owed from third parties to the practice. The practice will have completed this work within the accounting period but not yet received payment for it. For example, medical reports may have been written and sent to solicitors, but the income may not be received until after the year-end.

Depreciation
The reduction in the value of an asset due to wear and tear is measured by what is known as depreciation. Depreciation is a way of 'writing off' the cost of the asset over its useful economic life. Depreciation is shown as an expense in the profit and loss account each year.

Gross profit
For a trading business which buys goods at one price and then sells the same goods at a higher price, gross profits represent the difference between the two costs.

Liabilities
Liabilities are amounts that the practice owes. For example, the mortgage for the premises is a liability, as it is owed to the lender.

Net book value
The net book value is the original cost of the asset less the depreciation that has been charged to date. The net book value is an estimate of the value of the asset if sold at the accounting year-end.

Net equity
This is the difference between the value of the premises and the balance outstanding on the mortgage. If a practice is in negative equity, it means that its mortgage is higher than the value of the premises.

Net profit
The net profit is the final profit that the business has made, after deducting from the income all the expenses incurred (in running the business).

Overheads
Overheads are the expenses that are incurred in the day-to-day running of the practice; for example, salaries and wages of the practice staff.

Profit allocation
The partners in the practice are entitled to a share of profits; this is the net profit they have earned for the period. The profit allocation shows how the net profit for the period is shared amongst the partners.

Profit and loss
The profit and loss account (sometimes known as the income and expenditure account) shows the income, expenses and net profit for a given time period.

Profit sharing ratios
The profit sharing ratios (PSRs) are the ratios in which the partners in a partnership share the net profit.

Tangible assets

These will be the premises (if owned), fixtures, fittings, and office and medical equipment. The value of the premises on the balance sheet may be represented by either the original cost to purchase or build the property, or the open market value of the property. The open market value is the value that the practice would receive if the premises were sold.

Index

Major sections or chapters are highlighted in **bold**. Glossary entries are shown in *italics*.